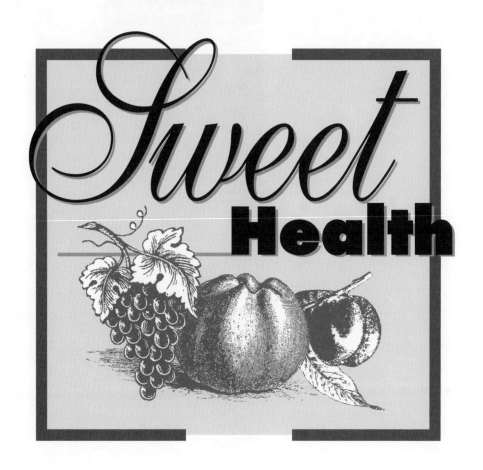

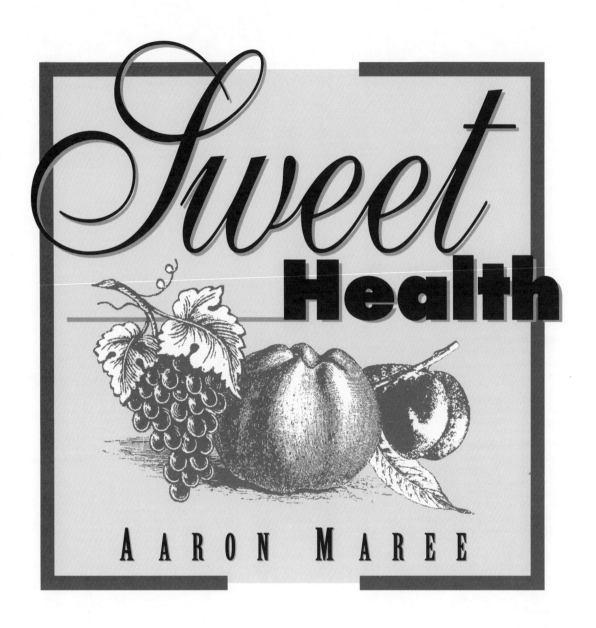

Sweet Health

AARON MAREE

Angus&Robertson
An imprint of HarperCollins*Publishers*

Angus&Robertson
An imprint of HarperCollins*Publishers*, Australia

First published in Australia in 1995

Text copyright © Maree Enterprises Pty Ltd 1995
Photographs copyright © HarperCollins*Publishers*

HarperCollins*Publishers*
25 Ryde Road, Pymble, Sydney NSW 2073, Australia
31 View Road, Glenfield, Auckland 10, New Zealand
77–85 Fulham Palace Road, London W6 8JB, United Kingdom
Hazelton Lanes, 55 Avenue Road, Suite 2900, Toronto, Ontario M5R 3L2
and 1995 Markham Road, Scarborough, Ontario, M1B 5M8, Canada
10 East 53rd Street, New York NY 10022, USA

National Library of Australia Cataloguing-in-Publication data:

Maree, Aaron
  Sweet health.

  ISBN 0 207 8428 3.
  Includes index.
  1. Confectionery. 2. Desserts. 3. Low-fat diet — Recipes. 4. Salt-free diet — Recipes.
  5. Low-cholesterol diet — Recipes. 6. Diabetic diet — Diet therapy — Recipes.
  7. Milk-free diet — Recipes. 8. Gluten-free diet — Recipes.
  I. Title.
641.563

Printed in Hong Kong

9 8 7 6 5 4 3 2 1
98 97 96 95

Photographs: Andre Martin
Front cover photograph: Blackberry Pots with Marinated Berries (page 27)
Back cover photograph: Moist Almond Torte (page 78)

CONTENTS

Introduction
7

Low-cholesterol
Desserts
9

Desserts for People
with Diabetes
28

Fat-free and
Low-fat Desserts
50

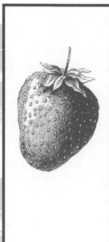

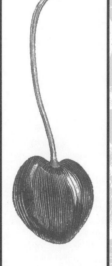

Gluten-free
Desserts
70

Lactose-free
Desserts
88

Salt-free and
Low-salt Desserts
108

Index
127

Dedication

Long before the idea for this book ever came to fruition, I had known people who were unable to eat the food that I adored so much, because of diabetes or other food intolerances. My childhood mentor and guide through life, our neighbour Tom Lee, a diabetic, was one of these. I felt this was terribly unfair.

Now that I have the opportunity to publish cookbooks, I decided to write this book for diabetics, coeliacs and other people with food intolerances, so that they can enjoy the food that I create.

Unfortunately, Tom Lee, the inspiration for this book, is no longer with us. However, my memories of him continue to inspire me in my life. I hope to produce many more works that would have made him proud.

'... At the going down of the sun, and in the morning
We will remember them.'

Laurence Binyon (1869–1943)

INTRODUCTION

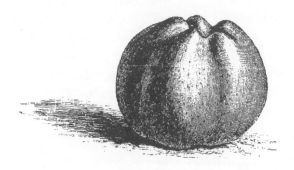

This book is not meant as a *weight loss guide.* Through my life and career I have always wondered what was so important about weight loss and having a trim figure. To me, personal happiness, the freedom to enjoy what we want when we want it — and, therefore, the choice to have either a large or a small body — is one of the few truly personal choices in life!

My choice was to be a pastry chef with extravagant tastes in food, a way of life in which being skinny is not even a consideration — as they say, 'you can't trust a skinny chef'. Of course in reality you can, and it must be said that even I have learnt a few things about health, weight-related problems and the physical hassles of being a larger person over the past two decades. Most of us now realise that in moderation, and combined with a sensible exercise program, almost everything is all right for you.

More to the point, though, this book is a

guide for those who have various ailments and intolerances and who are unable to enjoy many of food's sweet luxuries.

Every year I travel the world bringing pleasure to gourmets who enjoy the sweeter side of life and who feast on my creations of pastry, chocolate and sugar. It saddens me when in a class or lecture I meet someone who has come along to learn but is unable to eat the food because of intolerances to some products I have cooked with.

In everyday eating we all eat foods which are free of salt, free of gluten, fat and dairy products, etc. and we do not think anything of it. However, these foods are in fact the last bastions of hope for those who suffer from food allergies, intolerance or conditions such as diabetes.

Discovering that you have a food allergy or an intestinal disorder which makes your body reject certain food products is tough. Perhaps the best way to handle such news is to take the same approach that many dieters use: 'Think more of what it is you CAN eat, instead of what you can no longer eat.'

'Sweet Health' is a collection of recipes which fit the health guidelines for certain ailments and intolerances, bringing a positive approach to food for those who cannot eat everything they may desire. For all of us, a positive approach to desserts is a healthy approach to life.

For those who do not suffer from such ailments, the recipes in this book are just as delicious as any other desserts. You can use them for yourself and your family and friends. And who knows, one day you may really need to cook for someone with one of these dietary regimens. Also, if you are watching your weight or are on a diet, many of these recipes are especially suitable for you.

The majority of us are given complete freedom to choose a culinary lifestyle. I have chosen one of indulgent foods. To those who are not so fortunate and must follow a diet regimen, these recipes and my best wishes for a healthy, happy life are dedicated.

Low-cholesterol Desserts

Cholesterol is a type of fat. It is a waxy, white, fatty substance produced naturally by the body (daily, in the liver). Cholesterol also comes from the food we eat.

While some cholesterol is necessary for the body, if there is too much in the blood-stream, it builds up in the arteries (this is called atherosclerosis), narrowing the arteries and making it harder for the heart to pump blood around the body. This can lead to heart disease and possible heart attacks. Too much cholesterol in the bile can lead to gall stones.

The causes of high levels of blood cholesterol are eating too much saturated fat, being overweight and eating foods that are high in dietary cholesterol. Some people may inherit a predisposition to cholesterol problems.

The cholesterol story, which is often misunderstood and/or misquoted, can turn into a very complex scientific discussion, but for our purposes it is just a story about three major types of fats:

• Saturated fats are normally found in animal products and in certain vegetable fats. They are usually firm to hard at room temperature, e.g. fat on meat, skin on chicken, full cream dairy products, coconut and palm oil, high-fat snack foods and takeaways and commercially produced cakes and biscuits. These are the worst types of fat for cholesterol.
• Polyunsaturated fats can sometimes help reduce cholesterol if meals are also low in the saturated fats. They are found in some margarines and oils (such as safflower).
• Monounsaturated fats are found in nuts, margarines, seeds and some oils (such as olive oil), and are the 'good' fats, as they, like polyunsaturated fats, help lower cholesterol levels.

Foods that are high in dietary cholesterol should only be eaten occasionally — egg yolks, prawns and liver, for instance. Decreasing your intake of saturated fats reduces the chance of raising your cholesterol level.

Some foods labelled cholesterol-free can still be high in saturated fats and calories (e.g. certain oils can be high in fat but free of cholesterol, and prawns are high in cholesterol but free of fat).

The recipes in this chapter can be eaten by people who are on cholesterol-free diets. Also, if you have a high cholesterol count and need to lower it, ask a physician or dietitian to advise you about what you should or should not eat. These desserts can also play a part in this kind of diet.

Berry and Mango Brulée

In a small bowl, mix the yoghurt with the honey. Refrigerate till required.

Peel the mangoes and finely slice the flesh of two of them. Purée the flesh of the third.

Wash the strawberries and blueberries and purée a third of the total quantity.

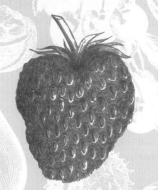

INGREDIENTS

3 cups (750 mL, 24 fl oz) plain low-fat yoghurt

3 teaspoons honey

3 whole ripe mangoes

200 g (6½ oz) fresh strawberries

200 g (6½ oz) fresh blueberries

90 g (3 oz) caster (superfine) sugar

fresh mint, for serving

Fill 6 soufflé ramekins, in the following order, until all the mixture is used up: fresh berries, mango purée, berry purée, mango slices, yoghurt and honey mixture. Chill the ramekins. Just before serving sprinkle some sugar on top of each ramekin. Place them under a grill or use a gas gun (torch) to caramelise the sugar into a golden brown toffee.

Allow 30 seconds for the sugar crust to set, then serve immediately, garnished with fresh mint.

Serves 6

Sienna Cake

Preheat the oven to 160°C (325°F). Line the base of a 20 cm (8 in) springform cake tin with non-stick baking parchment.

Place the honey, golden syrup and brown sugar in a saucepan and slowly bring to the boil. Boil, stirring continuously, for 5 minutes.

In a large mixing bowl, mix the flour, cocoa, cinnamon, fruits and nuts, lemon and orange zest and marmalade.

Pour the boiled mixture onto the fruit and nut mixture and stir until combined.

Pour the mixture into the prepared pan and press flat with the back of the spoon. Bake in the preheated oven for 25 minutes.

Remove the cake from the oven and dust it heavily with icing sugar while it is still hot.

½ cup (185 g, 6 oz) clear honey

¼ cup (90 g, 3 oz) golden syrup (light treacle)

1⅓ cups (225 g, 7 oz) brown sugar (light)

½ cup (60 g, 2 oz) plain (all-purpose) flour

½ cup (60 g, 2 oz) sifted cocoa powder

2 teaspoons ground cinnamon

1 cup (125 g, 4 oz) dried apricots, finely chopped

½ cup (90 g, 3 oz) glacé pineapple, chopped

1 cup (155 g, 5 oz) mixed (candied) peel

1½ cups (185 g, 6 oz) finely chopped hazelnuts (filberts)

1⅓ cups (155 g, 5 oz) finely chopped blanched almonds

¾ cup (90 g, 3 oz) finely chopped macadamia (Queensland) nuts

zest of 1 lemon

zest of 1 orange

1 tablespoon marmalade

icing (powdered) sugar, for dusting

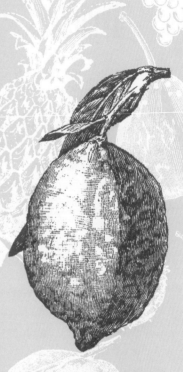

Let it cool, then store it for 24 hours. Cut it into very thin slices to serve with coffee.

Makes 20 to 30 thin slices

Crumble-topped Honey Pears

Preheat the oven to 180°C (325°F).

Heat the oil, honey and lemon juice and zest gently in a saucepan. Add the drained pears and heat slowly until warmed through.

Remove the pears from the saucepan. Place them flat side down in a casserole or deep pie dish and pour over any remaining liquid from the saucepan.

Combine the sponge crumbs, brown sugar, coconut and cinnamon and sprinkle over the pears.

Sprinkle the olive oil over the top of the crumble mixture and bake in the preheated oven for 25 minutes.

Serve warm.

Serves 4

INGREDIENTS

CRUMBLE-TOPPED HONEY PEARS

3 tablespoons olive oil

¼ cup (90 g, 3 oz) honey

juice and finely grated zest of 1 lemon

4 fresh pears, peeled, cored and halved, and soaked in lemon juice and water to prevent browning

1 cup (60 g, 2 oz) fresh sponge (cake) crumbs

2 tablespoons brown sugar (light)

2 tablespoons flaked coconut

½ teaspoon cinnamon

100 mL (3½ fl oz) olive oil

APPLE FRITTERS

60 g (2 oz) fresh compressed yeast

2 cups (500 mL, 16 fl oz) beer

3 cups (360 g, 12 oz) plain (all-purpose) flour

1 teaspoon cinnamon

1½ teaspoons salt

3 green cooking (Granny Smith) apples

¾ cup (100 g, 3½ oz) plain (all-purpose) flour

⅔ cup (100 mL, 3½ fl oz) puréed cranberries or raspberries

Apple Fritters

In a large bowl, whisk the yeast into the beer until it has dissolved. Add the flour, cinnamon and salt and stir to a thick paste. Place the bowl in a warm position for 2 hours, or until it has doubled in bulk.

When you are ready to serve the fritters, heat the oil to 180°C (350°F).

Peel, core and cut each apple (on the horizontal) into three or four slices, each 1–1.5 cm (½–⅔ in) thick.

Dip these first into the extra flour and then into the beer batter, coating them evenly, then place them straight into the hot oil.

Cook the fritters till they are golden brown on both sides (3–4 minutes for each side), then place them on absorbent kitchen paper (paper towels) and leave to drain for several minutes. Place two fritters on each plate and serve with the puréed cranberry or raspberry.

**Makes 9 to 12 fritters
(Serves 4 to 6)**

Raspberry Muffins

Preheat the oven to 200°C (400°F). Lightly grease a 12-cup muffin pan with canola oil.

In a bowl, place the oat bran, rice bran and bicarbonate of soda and stir until well combined.

In a blender or food processor, purée half of the raspberries with the sugar, until smooth.

In another bowl, mix the purée, milk and oil, then stir in the dry ingredients, followed by the remaining raspberries.

Beat the egg whites until they form stiff peaks, then fold them into the batter. Spoon the mixture into the muffin tins and bake for 20 minutes. These muffins may be heavier than others, but they should be moist.

INGREDIENTS

1½ cups (185 g, 6 oz) oat bran

1 cup (125 g, 4 oz) rice bran

1 teaspoon bicarbonate of soda

500 g (1 lb) fresh raspberries

¼ teaspoon ground cinnamon

¼ cup (60 g, 2 oz) caster (superfine) sugar

½ cup (125 mL, 4 fl oz) skim milk

2 tablespoons canola oil

3 egg whites

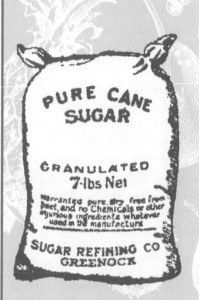

Variation
This recipe works just as deliciously with lightly stewed fruits such as apple, apricot and pear, with a little cinnamon, cloves or allspice for flavour.

Makes 12 muffins

Chocolate Cake

Preheat the oven to 180°C (350°F). Line the base of a 20 cm (8 in) cake tin with non-stick baking parchment.

In a bowl, combine the oat bran, flour, cocoa, baking powder and coffee liquid.

Whisk the egg whites until they form stiff peaks, then add the sugar, a spoonful at a time. Keep whisking until the sugar is incorporated and dissolved.

Fold half of the dry ingredients into the egg whites, then add the other half, folding until all the dry ingredients are incorporated. Try not to knock too much air out of the egg whites.

Pour the mixture carefully into the prepared cake tin. Bake for 40–45 minutes. Cool in the tin for 5 minutes then use a knife to loosen the cake from the tin and turn it onto a cake rack to cool.

INGREDIENTS

1 cup (125 g, 4 oz) oat bran

¼ cup (30 g, 1 oz) plain (all-purpose) flour

4 tablespoons unsweetened cocoa powder

½ teaspoon baking powder (soda)

2 teaspoons instant coffee granules, mixed with 1 tablespoon warm water

5 egg whites

1 cup (250 g, 8 oz) sugar

light mousse or fresh fruit coulis, for serving

Serve the cake in thin slices, either sandwiched with a light mousse or warmed and on a bed of fresh fruit coulis.

Serves 10

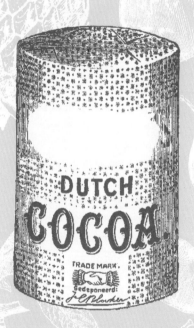

Light Lemon Cake

Drain and rinse the navy beans. Preheat the oven to 180°C (350°F). Line the base of a 20 cm (8 in) cake tin with non-stick baking parchment.

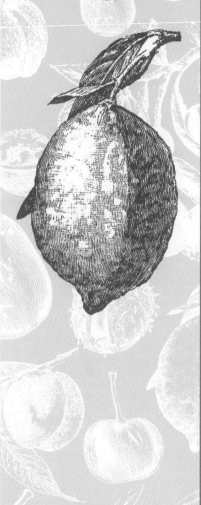

1½ cups (280 g, 9 oz) canned navy beans

⅔ cup (155 g, 5 oz) caster (superfine) sugar

4 tablespoons lemon juice

zest of 2 lemons, finely grated

¼ cup (30 g, 1 oz) rice bran

5 egg whites

In a blender or food processor, purée the beans with half the sugar and the lemon juice and zest, until smooth. Add the rice bran and purée again.

Whisk the egg whites until stiff peaks form, then add the sugar, a spoonful at a time. Keep whisking until the sugar is incorporated and dissolved.

Fold the egg white mixture into the bean mixture, then carefully (so as not to knock out any of the air from the mixture) pour it into the cake tin. Bake in the preheated oven for 45–50 minutes, or until the cake springs back when touched.

Serves 10

Cheesy Filo and Berry Stacks

Preheat the oven to 200°C (400°F).

Brush a single sheet of filo with egg white, top with another sheet and repeat this until all sheets are used up.

With a 5 cm (2 in) round scone (cookie) cutter, cut out discs of pastry and place them on a greased baking tray (sheet) lined with non-stick baking parchment. Cover with another sheet of non-stick baking parchment and top with another baking tray to ensure the discs stay flat.

Bake until golden brown, about 10–12 minutes. Leave the discs to cool on a wire rack.

In a bowl, combine the raspberries, blackberries and blueberries with the orange zest and juice. Refrigerate until required.

INGREDIENTS

8–10 filo (phyllo) pastry sheets

2 egg whites, lightly beaten

100 g (3½ oz) fresh raspberries

100 g (3½ oz) fresh blackberries

60 g (2 oz) fresh blueberries

finely grated zest and juice of 1 orange

1 cup (250 g, 8 fl oz) low-fat ricotta

1 tablespoon low-fat milk

¼ teaspoon cinnamon

1 tablespoon honey

1 large mango

1 tablespoon icing (powdered) sugar

fresh mint, for serving

In a small bowl, combine the ricotta, milk, cinnamon and honey. Refrigerate until well chilled, about 20–30 minutes.

To serve, take three discs for each plate and place them at 12, 4 and 8 o'clock.

Place a spoonful of the cheese mixture on each disc and top each with some of the berries. Top with another spoonful of the cheese mixture. Place a selection of the fresh berries on top of the cheese-covered disc stacks.

In a blender or food processor, purée the mango flesh until smooth. Spoon a small amount of purée into the centre of each plate and dust the entire plate with icing sugar.

Serve a sprig of fresh mint in the centre of each plate.

Serves 6

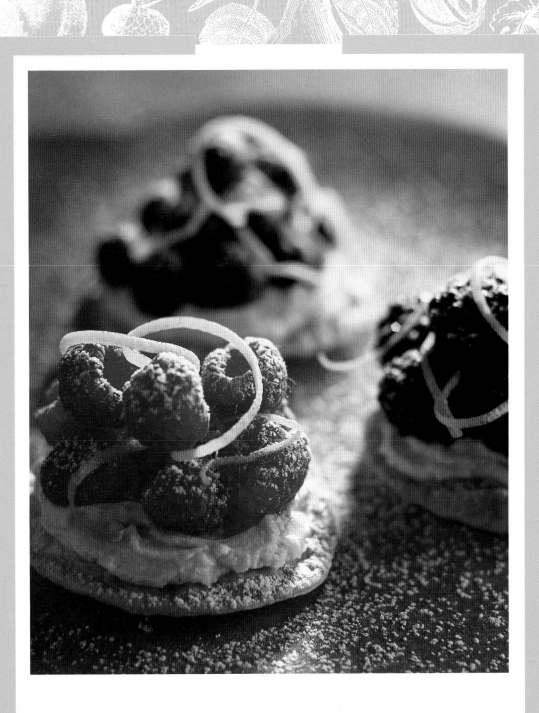

Cheesy Filo and Berry Stacks

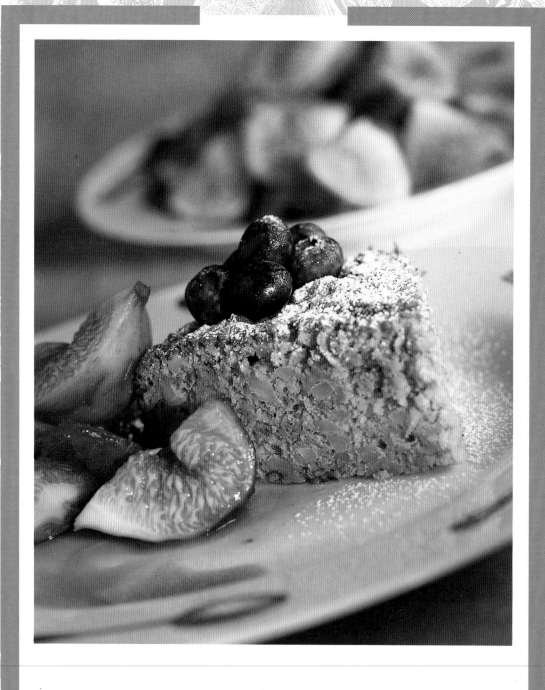

Almond, Apple and Zucchini Cake (front) and 'Pickled' Figs (behind)

'Pickled' Figs

Carefully peel the figs, so as not to cut through to the flesh, and place them in a deep casserole dish or pie dish. The tops of the figs should not come to the top of the dish.

Place the red wine, sugar, cinnamon sticks, cloves and the lemon halves in a saucepan and bring slowly to the boil. Simmer for 10 minutes.

Add the orange segments, orange zest and Grand Marnier to the wine liquid, then carefully pour the entire hot mixture over the figs. Let the mixture cool to room temperature, then cover and refrigerate for 24 hours.

Place the figs carefully on one serving platter and arrange the orange segments around them. Strain the remaining liquid and return it to a saucepan. Bring it to the boil, then continue boiling until it has reduced in volume by a third. Ladle this syrup over the figs and serve.

Serves 4

INGREDIENTS

'PICKLED' FIGS

8 fresh figs

2 cups (500 mL, 16 fl oz) red wine

⅓ cup (90 g, 3 oz) sugar

2 cinnamon sticks

2 cloves

1 lemon, cut in half

3 oranges, peeled and segmented

⅓ cup orange zest, cut into julienne

2 tablespoons Grand Marnier

ALMOND, APPLE AND ZUCCHINI CAKE

½ cup (60 g, 2 oz) plain (all-purpose) flour

½ cup (60 g, 2 oz) oat bran

1 cup (125 g, 4 oz) rice bran

1 teaspoon baking powder (soda)

½ teaspoon allspice

1 cup (125 g, 4 oz) chopped almonds

1 cup grated zucchini

1 cup grated apple

1 cup (250 mL, 8 fl oz) evaporated milk

4 egg whites

225 g (7 oz) sugar

icing (powdered) sugar and berry coulis, for serving

Almond, Apple and Zucchini Cake

Preheat the oven to 180°C (350°F). Line the base of a 20 cm (8 in) cake tin with non-stick baking parchment.

In a bowl, mix the flour, oat bran, rice bran, baking powder and allspice thoroughly.

Stir in the chopped almonds, grated zucchini and grated apple, followed by the evaporated milk.

Beat the egg whites until stiff peaks form. While still whisking, add the sugar, a spoonful at a time. Whisk until it is incorporated and dissolved. Fold the egg whites into the batter and pour it into the cake tin. Bake in the preheated oven for 1 hour, then let the cake cool in the pan. Be careful when removing the cake from its tin, as it is a very moist cake.

Dust lightly with icing sugar and serve (warm or cold) in slices with a rich berry coulis.

Serves 10

Cinnamon Orange Crisps

Preheat the oven to 180°C (350°F). Line two baking trays (sheets) with non-stick baking parchment.

In a bowl, combine the oat bran, flour, baking powder, cinnamon and orange zest.

In a separate bowl, mix the oil and glucose. Stir this into the dry ingredients (the mixture will be crumbly).

Whisk the egg whites until stiff peaks form, then add the sugar, a spoonful at a time. Keep whisking until the sugar is incorporated and dissolved.

Fold the egg whites into the dry mixture.

Place tablespoonfuls of the mixture, well apart, on the lined baking tray. Bake the cookies for 12–15 minutes, making certain they do not burn.

Makes 24

INGREDIENTS

CINNAMON ORANGE CRISPS

1 cup (125 g, 4 oz) oat bran

¾ cup (90 g, 3 oz) plain (all-purpose) flour

1 teaspoon baking powder (soda)

1 teaspoon cinnamon

finely grated zest of 1 orange

¼ cup (60 mL, 3 fl oz) olive oil

¼ cup (60 mL, 3 fl oz) liquid glucose (corn syrup)

2 egg whites

½ cup (90 g, 3 oz) brown sugar (light)

CHOCOLATE BROWNIES

1¾ cups (185 g, 6 oz) wholemeal (whole-wheat) plain flour

¾ teaspoon bicarbonate of soda

1 teaspoon baking powder (soda)

250 g (8 oz) fresh tofu

310 g (10 oz) honey

½ cup (125 mL, 4 fl oz) olive oil

¾ cup (100 g, 3½ oz) unsweetened cocoa powder

¾ cup (185 mL, 6 fl oz) water

½ cup (30 g, 1 oz) shredded coconut

¾ cup (90 g, 3 oz) chopped macadamia (Queensland) nuts

Chocolate Brownies

Preheat the oven to 180°C (350°F). Lightly grease a 23 cm (10 in) springform cake tin and line the base with non-stick baking parchment.

Sift the flour, bicarbonate of soda and baking powder into a bowl.

In another bowl, combine the tofu, honey, olive oil, cocoa and water. Add the sifted ingredients to this mixture, then stir in the coconut and the macadamia nuts.

Pour the mixture into the prepared pan and bake in the preheated oven for 35–40 minutes.

Let the brownies cool, then refrigerate them for 2–3 hours before serving.

Cut them into thin wedges to serve with coffee.

Makes 12 to 18

Carrot and Cardamom Bread

Preheat the oven to 180°C (350°F). Line the base of a loaf tin with non-stick baking parchment.

In a bowl, combine the carrot purée, cardamom seeds, sugar and the oil. Fold through the raisins.

In another bowl, mix together the oat bran, baking powder, and bicarbonate of soda.

Whisk the egg whites until they form stiff peaks, then add the extra sugar, a spoonful at a time. Keep whisking until the sugar is incorporated and dissolved.

Pour the liquid onto the dry ingredients. Place half of the egg whites on top. Fold these ingredients together to form a batter. Fold the remaining half of the egg whites into the mixture, then pour it into the lined loaf pan.

INGREDIENTS

1 cup carrot purée

1 tablespoon cardamom seeds

¾ cup (185 g, 6 oz) sugar

2 tablespoons olive oil

1 cup (155 g, 5 oz) raisins

2 cups (250 g, 8 oz) oat bran

½ teaspoon baking powder (soda)

¼ teaspoon bicarbonate of soda

3 egg whites

¼ cup (60 g, 2 oz) sugar, extra

Bake for 1 hour, then leave it to cool for 5 minutes in the tin before unmoulding. Let the bread cool completely, then slice it thinly and serve it as a savoury accompaniment to light savoury dishes or as an accompaniment to sweet mousses and other desserts.

Serves 10

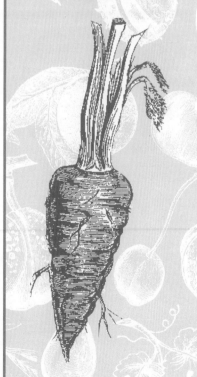

Steamed Figgy Pudding

Place the dried fruit, cinnamon and orange juice and zest in a saucepan, bring to the boil and allow to simmer for 5 minutes. Remove from the heat and cool.

Add the flour, baking powder, and egg white, and a little water or milk if necessary. Mix well.

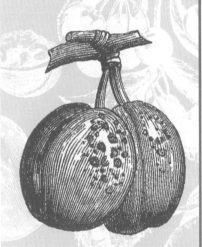

INGREDIENTS

1 cup (155 g, 5 oz)
dried pears

½ cup (90 g, 3 oz)
chopped dried figs

½ cup (90 g, 3 oz) sultanas

½ cup (90 g, 3 oz)
chopped dried apricots

½ teaspoon ground cinnamon

½ cup (125 mL, 4 fl oz)
unsweetened orange juice

zest of 2 oranges,
finely grated

1 cup (250 g, 4 oz)
wholemeal (whole-wheat)
plain flour

1½ teaspoons baking powder
(soda)

2 egg whites, beaten

fresh fruit, for serving

Lightly grease a 4 cup pudding basin with canola oil, then pour the mixture in.

Place a sheet of non-stick baking parchment onto an equal sized piece of aluminium foil. Fold the two sheets together across the centre so that a crease is formed. Place this crease over the top of the pudding basin (so it is central), with the baking parchment closest to the pudding, and fold the sides down tightly around the basin.

Place the pudding basin in a pot of boiling water. Cover the pot with a lid and boil (or steam) the pudding for 1 hour.

Serve small portions with fresh fruit.

Serves 4 to 6

Summer Pudding

Place the berries, sugar and orange juice in a saucepan. Bring slowly to the boil, then simmer gently for 5–6 minutes, until the berries begin to soften and break down. Do not let them turn to absolute pulp.

When the fruit has softened, remove the saucepan from the heat and let the mixture cool.

Line a 1.5 litre (2½ imp. pint) pudding bowl with three-quarters of the bread slices, then fill with the fruit mixture.

Carefully spoon the cooled fruit mixture into the bread lined bowl without allowing too much of the fruit's liquid into the bowl (reserve the remaining juice). Press the fruit down so it will all fit in.

Cover the top with the reserved bread slices, cutting them to fit if required.

INGREDIENTS

900 g (2 lb) mixed berries: redcurrants, blueberries, blackberries, raspberries

⅓ cup (90 g, 3 oz) sugar

90 mL (3 fl oz) orange juice

zest of 2 oranges, coarsely grated

10 slices fresh or day-old (low-fat) bread, crusts removed

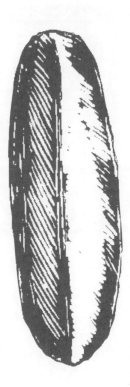

Pour over the reserved fruit juice, and let it soak into the bread and fruit slowly, then place a sheet of baking parchment and a flat plate or lid on top of the pudding and weigh it down using a foil-covered rock, some food tins or a 1 kg (2 lb) weight.

Refrigerate the pudding for 1–2 days, then remove it from the refrigerator and take off the weights and flat plate or lid. Run a thin knife around the outside edge of the pudding and then invert it onto a large plate. Give the mould a sharp shake if the pudding will not come out.

Serves 6 to 8

Passionfruit Soufflé

Preheat the oven to 180°C (350°F).

Place the sugar, water and passionfruit pulp in a saucepan and bring to the boil. Boil the mixture to soft ball stage (116–118°C/ 240–245°F), then let it cool.

Whisk the egg whites until stiff peaks form, then add the extra sugar, a spoonful at a time. Keep whisking until the sugar is dissolved.

Fold 2–3 tablespoons of the passionfruit purée through the egg whites. Store the rest in the refrigerator for use later. The total amount of passion-fruit pulp will make enough soufflé for 8–10 people.

Pour the mixture into a soufflé dish which has been lightly oiled with canola oil. Level off the soufflé at the top of the dish.

Bake in the preheated oven for 12 minutes, then dust lightly with icing sugar and serve immediately.

Serves 2

INGREDIENTS

PASSIONFRUIT SOUFFLÉ

1¼ cups (310 g, 10 oz) sugar

1¼ cups (310 mL, 10 fl oz) water

1¼ cups (310 mL, 10 fl oz) fresh passionfruit pulp

3 egg whites

2 tablespoons sugar, extra

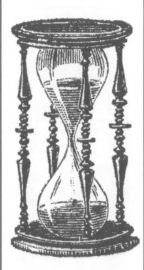

POMEGRANATE PARFAITS

1 tablespoon powdered gelatine

¼ cup (60 mL, 2 fl oz) cold water

½ cup (125 mL, 4 fl oz) fresh orange juice

2 tablespoons plain (all-purpose) flour

¾ cup pomegranate seeds

1 cup (250 mL, 8 fl oz) hot water

Pomegranate Parfaits

Mix the gelatine and cold water together.

Combine enough fruit juice with the flour to make a smooth paste. Add the remaining juice and the hot water. Place the liquid in a small saucepan and bring slowly to the boil, stirring continuously.

Lower the heat and add the gelatine. Stir until the gelatine has dissolved.

Remove the saucepan from the heat and let the mixture cool. Then refrigerate it. When it begins to set, whisk the mixture vigorously for 2–3 minutes, then fold through the pomegranate seeds.

Spoon into parfait glasses and return to refrigerator until set.

Sprinkle the tops with grated orange zest before serving.

Serves 4

Yoghurt, Apricot and Orange Mousse

INGREDIENTS

⅓ cup (90 mL, 3 fl oz) orange juice

⅓ cup (60 g, 2 oz) sago

2 tablespoons powdered gelatine

3 cups (750 mL, 24 fl oz) fresh orange juice, extra

475 g (15 oz) canned apricot halves

⅓ cup (90 mL, 3 fl oz) apricot juice from tin

1½ cups (310 g, 10 oz) fresh low-fat ricotta cheese

In the refrigerator, soak the sago in the orange juice overnight.

Dissolve the gelatine in the extra orange juice.

Place the sago and orange juice in a saucepan and bring to the boil, stirring continually until the sago is clear. Add the gelatine and stir to dissolve, then remove from the heat and leave to cool.

In a blender or food processor, blend the apricots with 3–4 tablespoons of the apricot juice until smooth. Add the ricotta and blend.

Fold the fruit mixture into the sago mixture and pour into a wet 6 cup ramekin or serving dish. Leave the mixture in the refrigerator overnight, to set, then serve with fresh fruit.

Serves 6

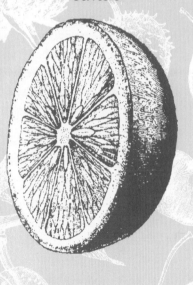

'Snow Top' Fruit Pie

Preheat the oven to 180°C (350°F). Lightly grease a deep 20 cm (8 in) quiche dish (pie dish).

Place the sugar and water in a saucepan and bring to the boil. Add the chopped apple, rhubarb, pear and lemon juice and zest. Reduce the heat and simmer gently with the lid on for 10 minutes, or until the fruit is tender when stabbed with a knife or toothpick.

Whisk the egg whites until soft peaks form, then add the sugar, a little at a time, and continue whisking until the sugar has dissolved. Sprinkle on the almonds and coconut, then fold through. Spread the meringue over the fruit.

INGREDIENTS

¾ cup (185 g, 6 oz) sugar

½ cup (125 mL, 4 fl oz) water

2 medium sized apples, peeled, cored and cut into 1 cm (½ in) dice

2 cups (301 g, 10 oz) chopped rhubarb

1 medium sized pear, peeled, cored and cut into 1 cm (½ in) dice

juice and zest of 1 lemon, finely grated

MERINGUE TOPPING

3 egg whites

3 tablespoons sugar

1 tablespoon flaked almonds

1 tablespoon shredded coconut

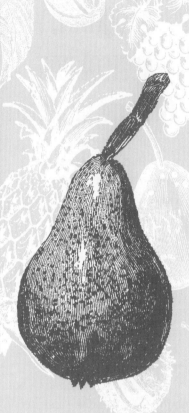

Bake in the preheated oven for 10–15 minutes, or until the meringue crust is golden brown and crisp.

Serve immediately.

Serves 6 to 8

Blackberry Pots with Marinated Berries

This rich dessert treat is a variation of a dessert I once served to a medical convention in England. It is best made during the height of the berry season, as it tends to be an expensive dish otherwise.

In a blender or food processor, blend the thawed berries and their juice with the yoghurt, sugar and gelatine.

Place the mixture in a saucepan and bring slowly to the boil, stirring constantly. Reduce the heat and simmer for 2–3 minutes, then remove the saucepan from the heat and let the mixture cool.

Place two fresh blackberries in the base of each of 8–10 250 mL (1 cup) ramekin dishes. Pour the mixture into the ramekins and refrigerate overnight.

3⅓ cups (850 g, 28 oz) frozen blackberries, thawed (retain the juice as they thaw)

1½ cups (250 g, 8 oz) non-fat yoghurt

½ cup (125 g, 4 oz) sugar

2½ tablespoons powdered gelatine

20 fresh blackberries

MARINATED BERRIES

½ cup (125 mL, 4 fl oz) water

juice and zest of 2 oranges

¼ cup (60 g, 2 oz) sugar

500 g (1 lb) mixed berries (strawberries, raspberries, blackberries and blueberries)

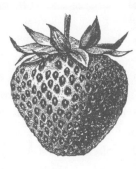

Serve with the marinated berries, a sprig of mint and two Cinnamon Orange Crisps (see page 20) at the side of each dish.

MARINATED BERRIES

Place the water, orange juice and zest and sugar in a saucepan and bring to the boil. Simmer gently for 2–3 minutes.

Add the berries and cook for a further 1 minute, then remove from the heat and refrigerate until cold.

Serves 8 to 10

DESSERTS FOR PEOPLE WITH DIABETES

As a child I was shattered to find that one of my dear friends, after being diagnosed as having diabetes, would no longer be able to live the carefree eating and drinking lifestyle he had led before. At such a young age I could not understand the complexity of what he had, but as I grew older I still felt it was unfair that he could not eat the same foods that I enjoyed and sometimes could not eat what I did as often as I could.

This book came about because of this one man. In the two decades since he was diagnosed, the lifestyles of people with diabetes have been improved greatly because of better health care and treatment. However, there is still no cure for the thousands of people with diabetes worldwide.

Diabetes is caused by the body's inability to make proper use of the sugars and starches that are consumed because of an inadequate production of insulin. Insulin is a hormone that is produced in the pancreas. It enables the body's cells to absorb glucose, the main fuel source used by the body.

In people with diabetes, either the pancreas makes too little insulin, or the insulin produced is unable to be effective. The latter is particularly likely in people who are overweight.

The sugars and starches we eat are turned into glucose in the small intestine. The glucose is then absorbed into the bloodstream. More insulin is produced by the pancreas in response to this rise in blood glucose. The insulin then helps to keep blood glucose levels under control by helping this extra glucose be absorbed by the body's tissues. If there is not enough insulin, or the insulin produced is ineffective, this extra glucose stays in the blood, causing levels to rise. This causes the symptoms of diabetes.

The most common symptoms are increased tiredness, increased frequency of urination and excessive thirst.

Diabetes may be controlled through diet and exercise. Some people may require tablets and a few may require injections of insulin. People with diabetes need to be particularly careful with their intake of fats, especially animal fats, because they are more at risk of blood vessel disease than other people, and therefore are more prone to heart attacks and strokes.

The recipes created for the sugar-free section of this book use two basic types of sugar substitutes — liquid and powdered. They are used according to their varying reactions to heat, their taste and their aroma. You will find most of the available sugar replacements in your local supermarket, local pharmacy or drugstore and if you have diabetes, you have probably already sampled most of these to test their sweetness, aftertaste and aroma, and see which you prefer.

The other important point for people with diabetes, especially those who are only newly diagnosed, to remember when shopping for everyday foods, is that sugar is called many different names on packet labels. These names include: carbohydrate, cane sugar, glucose, fructose, honey, malt, molasses, maple syrup, golden syrup, treacle, sugar beet and lactose. All labels should therefore be checked.

The more common suitable artificial sweeteners found in foods and drinks are aspartame (Nutrasweet), acesulphame K, cyclamate, saccharin, sucralose (Splenda) and Isomalt.

As these sweeteners are intensely sweet, they should be used sparingly. Some have aftertastes and aromas, some perform better in cold products, and some perform best in baked goods. For the recipes in this book we have taken all these factors into consideration, and therefore recommend that you use the suggested sugar replacement.

The recipes have been chosen for their diversity and because they are recipes I enjoy. Each has been carefully tested to conform with healthy low fat and low added sugar guidelines. I have restricted most recipes to 10 g fat and 15 g carbohydrates per serving.

In several cases the recipes have strayed slightly beyond these guidelines, but care with limiting fat intake over the day will mean that these desserts can still be served, as a pleasant change to the diet.

If you have diabetes, you should have your diet assessed by a dietitian, who will take into account not only your food likes and dislikes, but also your exercise and other daily life patterns.

If you are unsure about the types and amounts of foods you can enjoy, ask your local doctor for a referral to a dietitian or a diabetes centre.

Akwadu Pancakes

'Akwadu' is a favourite African dessert consisting of coconut and bananas cooked together. This delicious variation combines those same moist and subtle flavours in pancakes.

Place the dry ingredients in a bowl. Mash the banana with the lemon juice and add to the dry ingredients. Add the egg and coconut milk and combine thoroughly.

Grease a frypan (skillet) with a little oil, then heat it. Don't overheat the pan or the mixture will splatter. Use 3 tablespoons of batter per pancake. Cook each pancake for a few minutes on each side, or turn after bubbles appear in the top of the mixture.

INGREDIENTS

1 cup (125 g, 4 oz) wholewheat (whole-meal) plain flour

½ teaspoon baking powder (soda)

½ teaspoon cinnamon

pinch ground ginger

2 tablespoons skim milk powder

1 tablespoon powdered sweetener

1 medium banana

1 tablespoon lemon juice

1 egg (55 g, 2 oz)

⅓ cup (75 mL, 2½ fl oz) unsweetened coconut milk

2 teaspoons polyunsaturated vegetable oil, for greasing

Serves 6

CHO – 15.8 g
FAT – 5.8 g
KJ – 561
CALS – 133.5

The cholesterol in this recipe is slightly above the recommended amount.

Vanilla Custards

Preheat the oven to 170°C (340°F).

Heat the milk with the vanilla pod until the milk boils, then stir in the sweetener. Remove from the heat.

Beat the yolks until thick and pale in colour, then add the milk, stirring constantly. Remove the vanilla pod, split it and place the seeds back in the mixture.

Strain the custard mixture before pouring it into 5 ½ cup moulds or ramekins. Sprinkle with the cinnamon. Set them in a baking tray, and pour in enough hot water to reach halfway up the sides of the moulds. Cover the whole baking tray with foil and bake for about 1 hour, or until set.

INGREDIENTS

2 cups (500 mL, 16 fl oz) skim milk

1 teaspoon liquid sweetener

1 vanilla pod

3 egg yolks (65 g, 2 oz eggs)

¼ teaspoon cinnamon

Remove the moulds from the water bath. Let them cool, then refrigerate them. Serve chilled.

Serves 5

CHO – 5 g
FAT – 3.5 g
KJ – 302
CALS – 72

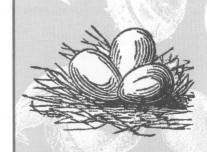

Frozen Citrus Soufflé

Take a large soufflé ramekin (5–6 cup) and wrap a band of non-stick baking parchment (double thickness) around the outside of the ramekin. Make sure it comes 10 cm (4 in) above the edge of the dish. Hold the band to the outside of the ramekin with rubber bands or string.

Soften the gelatine in the cold water.

Place the egg yolks in a saucepan with the sweetener, lemon and orange zest and the orange juice.

Heat, stirring constantly, until the mixture is thick. Do not let the mixture boil. Remove from the heat and add the softened gelatine, stirring to dissolve. Chill in the refrigerator until the mixture begins to thicken.

INGREDIENTS

1½ tablespoons powdered gelatine

½ cup (125 mL, 4 fl oz) cold water

8 medium eggs, separated

2 tablespoons powdered sweetener

finely grated zest of 1 lemon

finely grated zest of 1 orange

1 cup (250 mL, 4 fl oz) orange juice

½ cup (125 g, 4 oz) low-fat natural yoghurt

orange and lemon zest, for serving

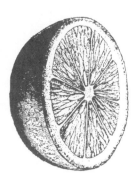

Remove from the refrigerator, then add the yoghurt and beat until well combined.

Whisk the egg whites in a clean bowl until they form stiff peaks. Carefully fold the egg whites into the yoghurt mixture. Gently spoon into the soufflé dish.

Place the soufflé in the freezer for 3 hours or longer. Before serving, remove the band of baking parchment. Serve with fresh orange and lemon zest.

Serves 10

CHO – 2.74 g
FAT – 4.52 g
KJ – 386.3
CALS – 92

Ice Cream

In this recipe, make sure that the gelatine mixture does not set before it is mixed with the other ingredients, otherwise the ice cream will not be smooth. Thirty minutes is normally sufficient time for freezing. It is advisable to stir the ice cream once or twice while it is freezing.

Dissolve the gelatine in the hot water with the sweetener.

Mix the milk with the cream and salt.

When the gelatine mixture is starting to cool, but is still liquid, add it to the milk mixture along with the vanilla.

Whisk the egg whites until they form stiff peaks, then fold them through the cream mixture.

Pour into an ice cream tray and freeze.

4 teaspoons powdered gelatine

4 tablespoons hot water

2 tablespoons powdered sweetener

140 mL (4½ fl oz) milk

100 mL (3½ fl oz) double (heavy, thickened) cream

pinch of salt

1 teaspoon vanilla extract, or to taste

2 egg whites

1 punnet strawberries, washed and hulled, for serving

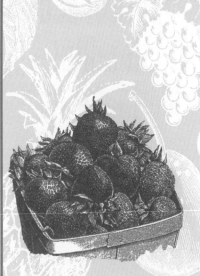

Remove from the freezer about 10 minutes before serving, then serve with fresh strawberries.

Serves 4

CHO – 3.8 g
FAT – 10.4 g
KJ – 604
CALS – 143.8

The fat content of this recipe is slightly above the recommended amount.

Apricot and Hazelnut Meringue Slice

½ cup (60 g, 2 oz)
plain (all-purpose) flour

¾ cup (60 g, 2 oz)
rolled (minute) oats

435 g (14 oz) can apricot
halves in natural juice,
drained (reserve 6
tablespoons of the juice)

2 eggs, separated

2 tablespoons
diet apricot jam

¼ teaspoon ground cinnamon

¾ cup (125 g, 4 oz)
ground roasted hazelnuts

2 tablespoons
shredded coconut

Preheat the oven to 180°C (350°F). Grease a 23 x 18 x 2 cm (9 x 7 x 1 in) baking tray (sheet) and line it with non-stick baking parchment.

In a blender or food processor blend the flour, rolled oats, 4 tablespoons of the reserved apricot juice and the egg yolks until well combined. Press into the base of the tin.

Blend the apricots and jam with the cinnamon until smooth, then spread this mixture over the base.

Beat the egg whites until they form stiff peaks, then fold in the finely ground hazelnuts, the remaining 2 tablespoons of apricot juice and the coconut. Spoon the mixture over the apricots.

Bake for 30–35 minutes. Cool, cut into bars and serve.

Makes 14

CHO – 9.53 g
FAT – 7.2 g
KJ – 487.35
CALS – 116

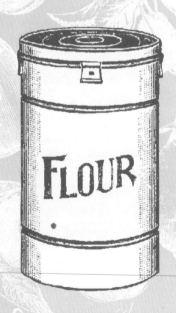

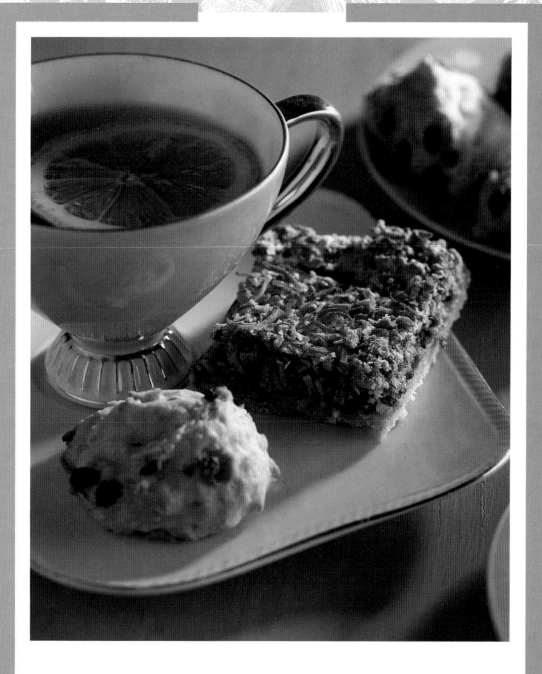

Apricot and Hazelnut Meringue Slice and Apple Cookies (page 42)

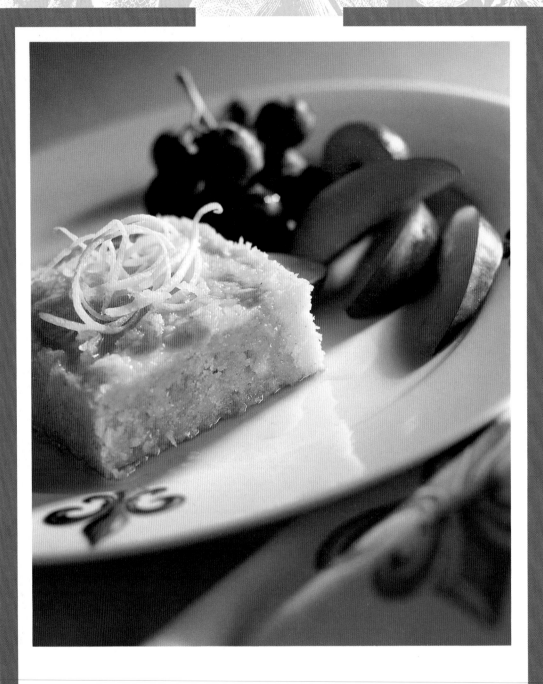

Lemon and Cardamom Syrup Cake (page 40)

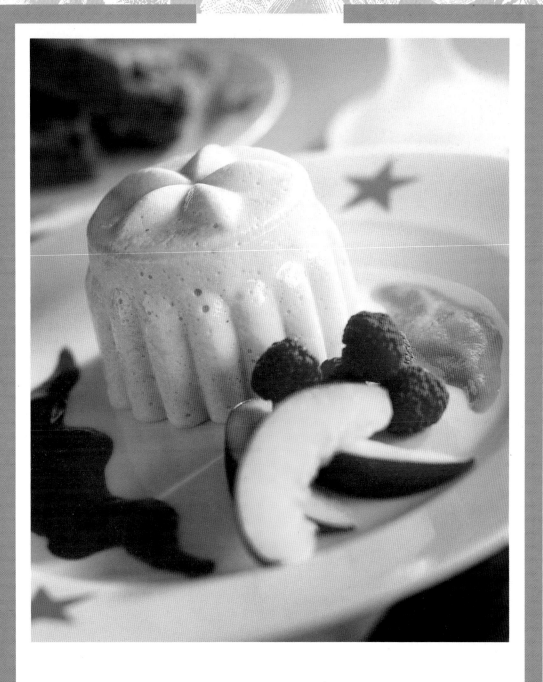

Apricot Mousse with a Symphony of Sauces (page 39)

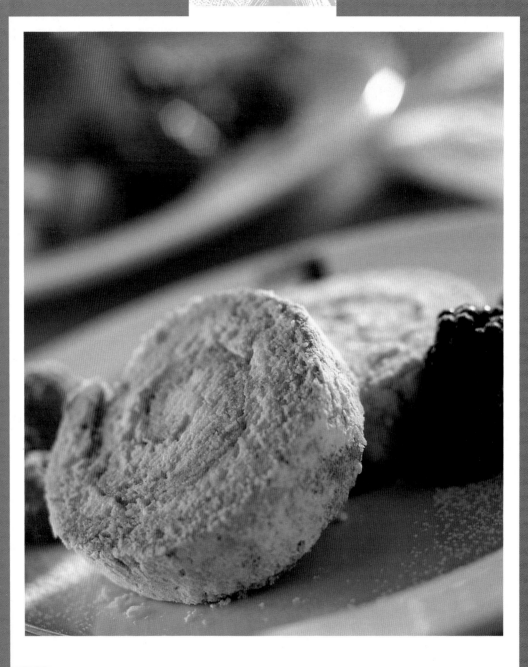

Light Tropical Roll (front, page 67) and Split Berry Bavarois (page 53)

Apricot Mousse with a Symphony of Sauces

INGREDIENTS

1½ tablespoons
powdered gelatine

5 tablespoons hot water

¼ cup (155 g, 5 oz)
dried apricots

100 g (3½ oz)
low-fat natural yoghurt

100 g (3½ oz)
ricotta cheese, sieved

2 egg whites

¾ cup (200 g, 6½ oz)
rockmelon, puréed

¾ cup (200 g, 6½ oz)
raspberries, puréed

fresh mint, to serve

Let the gelatine soak in the hot water.

Place the dried apricots in a large bowl and completely cover them with boiling water. Let them cool, then drain them completely. Repeat this process two more times.

Place the apricots in a blender or food processor with the yoghurt and ricotta and blend until smooth.

Place the soaked gelatine in a bowl and sit the bowl in some hot water until the gelatine dissolves. Add the gelatine to the apricot and yoghurt mixture and whisk in well.

Whisk the egg whites until they form soft peaks. Lightly fold the egg whites through the yoghurt mixture.

Evenly divide the mixture among six dariole moulds and refrigerate for 2–3 hours.

Unmould each mousse by dipping its base into hot water for several seconds. Place each unmoulded mousse in the centre of a serving plate.

Drizzle some rockmelon purée onto one side of each plate, and some raspberry purée onto the other side, around the mousse. Spread the purées using a spoon, and use a toothpick or skewer to swirl the two sauces together. Serve with a sprig of mint.

Serves 6

CHO – 15.6 g
FAT – 2.01 g
KJ – 513.5
Cals – 122.26

The cholesterol in this recipe is slightly above the recommended amount.

DESSERTS FOR PEOPLE WITH DIABETES

Lemon Cardamom Syrup Cake

Preheat the oven to 180°C (350°F).

Melt the margarine in a saucepan over a low heat. Stir in the jam, lemon juice and zest, water and eggs and whisk thoroughly to combine.

In a bowl, combine the flour, baking powder, bicarbonate of soda, cardamom and sweetener. Make a well in the centre of these, add the liquid ingredients and mix to combine.

Spoon the mixture into a greased 20 cm (8 in) square cake tin and bake in the preheated oven for 25–30 minutes, or until a toothpick inserted into the cake comes out clean.

INGREDIENTS

90 g (3 oz) margarine

2 tablespoons diabetic apricot jam

juice and zest of 2 lemons

2 tablespoons water

2 eggs

2 cups (250 g, 8 oz) plain (all-purpose) flour

1½ teaspoons baking powder (soda)

1 teaspoon bicarbonate of soda

½ teaspoon cardamom

½ cup (30 g, 1 oz) powdered sweetener

SYRUP

¼ cup (60 mL, 2 fl oz) water

¼ cup (15 g, ½ oz) powdered sweetener

finely grated zest of 2 lemons

juice of 1 lemon

SYRUP

Place all the ingredients in a saucepan and simmer over a medium heat for 2 minutes. Remove from the heat and spoon directly over the hot cake. Remove the cake from the tin after 5–10 minutes and let it cool on a cake rack.

Makes 15 slices

CHO – 12.1 g
FAT – 5.44 g
KJ – 450.73
CALS – 107.31

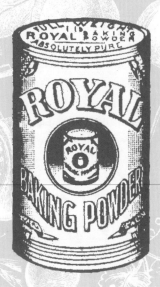

Deluxe Chocolate Brownies

Preheat the oven to 180°C (350°F).

In a saucepan, mix the cocoa with the hot water, until smooth. Add the butter and melt over a low heat. Remove from the heat and add the sweetener, vanilla and eggs. Beat until smooth.

Sift the flour and baking powder, then add them to the cocoa mixture and stir well. Add the walnuts.

Press the mixture into a 15 cm (6 in) square baking tin lined with non-stick baking parchment.

Bake the brownies for 20 minutes, then let them cool and cut them into fingers.

INGREDIENTS

3 tablespoons unsweetened cocoa powder, sifted

2 tablespoons hot water

90 g (3 oz) butter or margarine

2 teaspoons liquid sweetener

1 teaspoon vanilla extract

2 eggs (55 g), beaten

1 cup (125 g, 4 oz) plain (all-purpose) flour

1 teaspoon baking powder (soda)

¾ cup (30 g, 1 oz) chopped walnuts

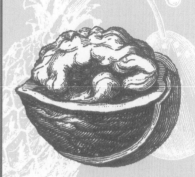

Makes 14

CHO – 7.2 g
FAT – 10.65 g
KJ – 566.85
CALS – 135

The fat content of this recipe is slightly above the recommended amount.

Apple Cookies

Preheat the oven to 190°C (375°F).

Sift the flour, salt, spices and baking powder together into a bowl.

In another bowl, beat the butter and sweetener until light and fluffy. Add the egg and combine well.

Add the sifted dry ingredients alternately with the apple purée, mixing well after each addition. Fold in the currants and bran cereal. Drop level tablespoons of the mixture (about 2 cm/1 in apart) onto a greased baking tray. Bake for 18 minutes, or until golden.

Makes 48

CHO – 5.3 g
FAT – 2.4 g
KJ – 188.8
CALS – 45

INGREDIENTS

APPLE COOKIES

1⅔ cups (225 g, 7 oz) plain (all-purpose) flour

1 teaspoon cinnamon

½ teaspoon ground cloves

1 teaspoon baking powder (soda)

125 g (4 oz) unsalted butter

2 teaspoons liquid sweetener

1 egg (60 g)

1 cup (250 mL, 8 fl oz) unsweetened apple purée (baby food is the best product to use for this)

⅓ cup (60 g, 2 oz) currants

½ cup (60 g, 2 oz) bran cereal

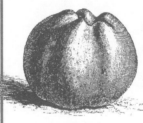

LEMON BUTTER

2¼ tablespoons unsalted butter

juice and zest of 2 medium lemons

1 egg (55 g), well beaten

1 tablespoon powdered sweetener

Lemon Butter

Stand a stainless steel bowl in a saucepan of boiling water. Chop the butter finely, place it in the bowl and let it melt.

Add the egg, lemon juice and zest and sweetener.

Stir continuously until the mixture thickens enough to coat the back of the spoon.

Let the mixture cool slightly, then strain and store in a jar for future use.

Lemon butter will keep in the refrigerator for 5–6 days.

NB: For a different flavour, or variations on this fabulous recipe, replace the lemon juice and zest with orange, grapefruit or lime.

Serve a small spoonful of these on selected desserts in place of cream.

Makes 155 mL (5 fl oz)

Analysis on total quantity
CHO – 3.1 g
FAT – 4.22 g
KJ – 1742
CALS – 415

English Breakfast Marmalade

Cut the zest from the oranges and lemons, without removing the white pith.

Chop the zest finely and place it in a large pot. Cut up the fruit flesh, weigh it, then add it and the water to the pot.

Bring slowly to the boil, then boil steadily for 30 minutes, until the flesh is soft and tender enough to break up with a spoon or whisk. Add the sweetener.

INGREDIENTS

2 oranges

3 lemons

2 cups (500 mL, 16 fl oz) water

2 tablespoons powdered sweetener

powdered gelatine

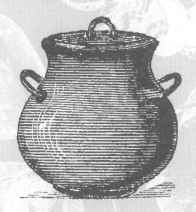

Add 1½ teaspoons of gelatine (dissolved in a little water) for every 250 g (8 oz) of pulp.

Remove the marmalade from the heat and bottle in sterilised jars while still hot. Let the marmalade cool in the jar(s) to room temperature, then store in the refrigerator. Gelatine is not a preservative, so make only enough jam for your immediate needs.

Makes approximately 1½ cups (310 g, 10 oz)

Analysis on total quantity
CHO – 9.5 g
FAT – 1.5 g
KJ – 347
CALS – 36

Chocolate Peanut Butter Cookies

Preheat the oven to 180°C (350°F). Line a baking tray (sheet) with non-stick baking parchment.

Place the sifted dry ingredients in a large bowl.

In a separate bowl mix the peanut butter with the remaining ingredients.

Add the dry ingredients to the peanut butter mixture and stir until combined thoroughly.

Drop teaspoonfuls onto the prepared tray, leaving 2–3 cm (1 in) between the spoonfuls.

Bake the cookies in the pre-heated oven for 20 minutes, then let them cool on the tray.

Makes 24

CHO – 1.65 g
FAT – 3.13 g
KJ – 194.79
CALS – 46.38

INGREDIENTS

CHOCOLATE PEANUT BUTTER COOKIES

¾ cup (90 g, 3 oz) soya flour, sifted

2 tablespoons unsweetened cocoa powder, sifted

1½ teaspoons baking powder (soda), sifted

⅓ cup (90 g, 3 oz) sugarless peanut butter

1 egg (55 g), beaten

2 teaspoons liquid sweetener

pinch of salt

½ cup (125 mL, 4 fl oz) skim milk

1 teaspoon vanilla extract

PUMPKIN ICE CREAM

2 cups (500 mL, 16 fl oz) cooked fresh pumpkin

5 eggs

2 cups (500 mL, 16 fl oz) skim milk

1 tablespoon fresh ginger, grated

1 teaspoon cinnamon

⅛ teaspoon allspice

⅓ cup (15 g, ½ oz) powdered sweetener

2 tablespoons Grand Marnier

Pumpkin Ice Cream

Combine all ingredients in a blender or food processor and purée till smooth and frothy.

Place the mixture in a large ramekin dish and freeze, stirring every 1 hour until frozen firm (4–5 hours altogether).

Remove from the freezer 15–20 minutes before serving, as it tends to freeze rather firm.

Makes 6 cups (1.5 litres, 3 pints), which serves 8

CHO – 10.4 g
FAT – 4 g
KJ – 488.8
CALS – 116.4

Strawberry Sherbet

In a blender or food processor, blend all the ingredients except the crushed ice. Then add the ice and blend until thickened. Serve immediately.

Serves 4

CHO – 10.3 g
FAT – 0.2 g
KJ – 329
CALS – 78.3

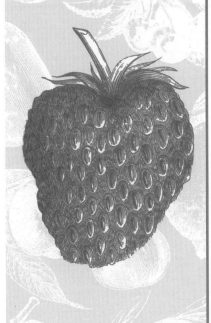

STRAWBERRY SHERBET

½ cup (125 g, 4 oz)
low-fat natural yoghurt

½ cup (125 mL, 4 fl oz)
skim milk

1 tablespoon
powdered sweetener

2 tablespoons
strawberry liqueur

1 teaspoon vanilla extract

1 cup (155 g, 5 oz)
fresh or frozen strawberries

1¼ cups crushed ice

APPLE, CHEESE AND COCONUT DELIGHT

1 cup wheatgerm

½ cup (45 g, 1½ oz)
desiccated (shredded)
coconut

½ cup (60 g, 2 oz) whole
almonds

60 g (2 oz) cottage cheese

800 g (26 oz) stewed apples
(approx. 1.3 kg, 1 lb 14 oz
fresh apples)

1 teaspoon liquid sweetener

2 teaspoons lemon rind

1 teaspoon cinnamon

½ cup flaked almonds

Apple, Cheese and Coconut Delight

Preheat the oven to 180°C (350°F). Line a 23 x 18 x 2 cm (9 x 7 x 1 in) baking tray (sheet) with non-stick baking parchment.

Blend the wheatgerm, coconut, almonds and cottage cheese in a blender or food processor.

Press this mixture into the lined baking tray.

Combine the apple, sweetener, lemon rind and cinnamon. Spread this mixture evenly over the base. Cover the top liberally with the flaked almonds.

Bake the slice until golden brown, about 20 minutes. Let the slice cool, then refrigerate it for 2–3 hours before cutting it into squares.

Makes 18 squares

CHO – 5.3 g
FAT – 5.9 g
KJ – 356.5
CALS – 84.9

Fruit Sensation

Preheat the oven to 190°C (375°F).

Lightly brush the sheets of pastry with the oil. Mix the spices together and evenly sprinkle the spice mix over the sheets.

Stack the sheets on top of each other and cut the stack into 3 pieces lengthwise and 4 horizontally, making 12 pieces.

Press the pieces into a 12 cup non-stick medium muffin pan to form baskets.

Bake for 6–8 minutes, or until golden brown. Let the muffin baskets cool, then carefully remove them from the pan.

Place a dollop of yoghurt into the base of each basket.

Toss the fruit together and pile some into each basket.

Cut the orange zest into thin strips. Place it in a saucepan with the orange juice,

INGREDIENTS

4 sheets filo (phyllo) pastry (50 x 28 cm, 20 x 11 in)

1 tablespoon vegetable oil

2 teaspoons cinnamon

1 teaspoon nutmeg

½ teaspoon cloves

FILLING

1 punnet small strawberries, washed, hulled and halved

2 ruby grapefruit, segmented, with segments cut in half

zest of 1 orange

100 mL (3½ fl oz) orange juice

2 tablespoons powdered sweetener

2 teaspoons powdered gelatine

½ cup (125 g, 4 oz) low-fat natural yoghurt

fresh mint, to garnish

sweetener and gelatine and heat gently until the gelatine has dissolved. Chill this syrup until it is partially set (10–15 minutes), then brush it over the fruit.

Garnish with the mint and serve.

Serves 12

CHO – 6.5 g
FAT – 1.9 g
KJ – 233.75
CALS – 55.65

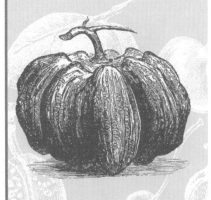

Individual Blueberry Pies

Preheat the oven to 200°C (400°F). Lightly brush the pastry sheets with oil and sprinkle the almonds on four of the sheets. Stack three of these four sheets on top of each other and place the plain sheet on top. Cut the pastry stack into 3 pieces lengthwise and 4 horizontally, making 12 pieces.

Press these into a 12-cup non-stick medium sized muffin pan to form baskets.

Fold the remaining sheet of filo in half and use a 4 cm (1½ in) fluted round cutter to cut out 12 lids. Place the lids on a baking tray (sheet) lined with non-stick baking parchment.

Bake the baskets and lids for 6–8 minutes, or until golden brown. Let them cool, then carefully remove baskets and lids from the pan and tray.

INGREDIENTS

5 sheets filo (phyllo) pastry (50 x 28 cm, 20 x 11 in)

1 tablespoon vegetable oil

¼ cup (15 g, ½ oz) ground almonds

FILLING

500 g (1 lb) fresh blueberries, washed

zest of 2 lemons, finely grated

2 teaspoons lemon juice

¼ teaspoon ground cloves

¼ teaspoon ground cinnamon

2 tablespoons powdered sweetener

2 teaspoons powdered gelatine

Place all the filling ingredients except the gelatine in a medium saucepan and simmer for 5–7 minutes. Remove from the heat and strain immediately. Place the berries in the refrigerator to cool. Add the gelatine to the remaining liquid while the liquid is still hot. Whisk to mix and dissolve, then chill the mixture until it is partially set.

Spoon the chilled berries into the pastry baskets, then spoon over the juice and top with the lids. Serve immediately.

Makes 12

CHO – 8.35 g
FAT – 3.17 g
KJ – 288
CALS – 68.57

Baked Apples

Preheat the oven to 180°C (350°F).

In a small bowl, combine the currants, cinnamon, breadcrumbs, almonds and sweetener. Add the egg white and mix thoroughly.

Halve the apples and scoop out the core, leaving a cavity. Place the apples on a baking tray and spoon the currant mixture into the cavities.

Bake the apples in the preheated oven for 30–35 minutes, then serve.

Serves 8

CHO – 10.86 g
FAT – 2.23 g
KJ – 293
CALS – 69.76

INGREDIENTS

BAKED APPLES

⅓ cup (60 g, 2 oz) currants

¼ teaspoon cinnamon

¼ cup (30 g, 1 oz) fresh breadcrumbs

¼ cup (30 g, 1 oz) ground almonds

½ teaspoon liquid sweetener

1 egg white

4 medium green cooking (Granny Smith) apples

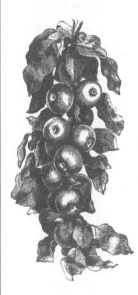

CITRUS PUDDINGS

4 eggs, separated

zest of 1 orange, finely grated

zest of 1 lemon, finely grated

1½ cups (375 mL, 12 fl oz) low-fat skim milk

⅓ cup (75 mL, 2½ fl oz) fresh orange juice

¼ teaspoon liquid sweetener

Citrus Puddings

Preheat the oven to 160°C (320°F).

Whisk the egg whites until they form stiff peaks.

In another bowl, whisk the egg yolks with the orange and lemon zest until light and fluffy. Add the milk and beat for a further minute. Add the orange juice and sweetener and combine thoroughly.

Fold the egg whites through the egg yolk mixture and spoon the mixture evenly into six small soufflé ramekins.

Place the ramekins in a baking tray and fill the tray with water so that it comes halfway up the sides of the ramekins. Bake in the preheated oven until the puddings are set, about 50 minutes. Let the puddings cool (out of the water bath) for 20 minutes before serving.

Serves 6

CHO – 4.28 g
FAT – 3.78 g
KJ – 328.16
CALS – 78.13

Lemon and Cinnamon Cookies

Preheat the oven to 180°C (350°F). Line a baking tray (sheet) with non-stick baking parchment.

Place the margarine, lemon zest and sweetener in a bowl and cream until light. Add the egg and mix in thoroughly.

Add the sifted flour, baking powder and cinnamon to the creamed mixture and mix. Add the milk and mix till just combined, to form a dough. Divide the dough into 24 balls.

Place the balls on the lined baking tray. Leave a small amount of room between them. Dip your thumb or a teaspoon into flour and press into the centre of each ball, to leave a small depression. Place a dot of apricot jam in each depression.

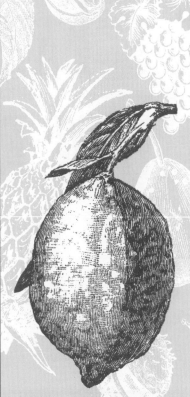

Bake in the preheated oven for 15–18 minutes, or until golden brown.

Makes 24

CHO – 7.8 g
FAT – 5.96 g
KJ – 376.95
CALS – 89.75

FAT-FREE AND LOW-FAT DESSERTS

Until researching this book, I, probably like many thousands of people, thought that eating a diet rich in fat literally meant that you stood the chance of becoming fat or overweight if your metabolism wasn't able to process these fats.

I now know that fat is a contributing factor in heart disease and heart attacks, high blood pressure, diabetes, hiatal hernias, strokes, gallstones and obesity, and that excess fat has been strongly linked to certain cancers.

While our bodies need fat, we get enough through normal healthy eating. So most of us, especially those who eat one or more meals of fast food a week, could afford to reduce our fat intake.

Fat helps the body maintain healthy skin and hair, it is a transporter of the fat-soluble vitamins — A, D, E and K — and it supplies fatty acids. It also gives us a feeling of satisfaction after a meal because it slows the emptying of food from the stomach.

The problem of being overweight is not solved by eradicating fat from the diet. One of the worst things we can do, other than abusing our bodies through excessive intake of fat and cholesterol, is to reverse this process and try dieting with an inadequate food plan. A low-fat high-fibre diet, usually supplied by a physician or dietitian, plus regular exercise, can help us maintain weight or lose weight as required.

Polish Sweet Koshav

This Polish dessert has a strong Jewish heritage. Its name comes from the word 'kosher', literally meaning 'allowed' or 'abiding by the kosher food laws'. This is a delicious dessert which gets better the longer it is left.

Place the currants, dried apricots, mixed peel, dates and raisins in a bowl and cover with cold water. Stir quickly and then drain.

Cover the fruit with boiling water (3–4 cups) and leave until the water becomes cold. Drain the fruit and set aside.

In a saucepan place the honey, orange segments, water, orange juice and zest, lemon juice and zest, cinnamon, cloves and allspice along with the fruit and chopped nuts.

125 g (4 oz) currants

155 g (5 oz) dried apricots, chopped

30 g (1 oz) mixed (candied) peel

90 g (3 oz) chopped dates

155 g (5 oz) raisins

¼ cup (90 g, 3 oz) honey

2 oranges, peeled and segmented

1½ cups (375 mL, 12 fl oz) water

1½ cups (375 mL, 12 fl oz) orange juice

zest of 2 oranges

zest and juice of 1 lemon

1 cinnamon stick

2 cloves

¼ teaspoon ground allspice

60 g (2 oz) macadamia (Queensland) nuts, lightly roasted and chopped

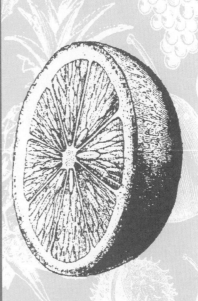

Bring slowly to the boil, over a gentle heat. Simmer for 20 minutes.

Remove from the heat and leave to cool. Refrigerate the cooled mixture overnight. Serve small bowls of the Koshav as a dessert, or serve it as an accompaniment to cake or any warm desserts.

Serves 4 to 6

FAT FREE AND LOW FAT DESSERTS

Zesty Lemon Torte

Preheat the oven to 200°C (400°F).

Lightly grease the sides of three 20 cm (8 in) cake tins. Line each base with a disc of non-stick baking parchment.

Whisk the egg whites until stiff peaks form, then gradually beat in the sugar, a spoonful at a time. Then beat at top speed on the mixer until the sugar is completely dissolved, about 5 minutes.

In another bowl, combine the almonds, cornflour and icing sugar, then use a spatula to very gently fold in the beaten egg whites.

Spoon a third of the mixture onto each disc. Spread the mixture evenly across the discs, staying inside the edge.

Bake the discs for 20 minutes then remove and allow to cool in the tins. Before they cool completely, run a sharp knife around the outside edge of each to loosen the disc from the tin. When the discs have cooled completely, and hardened, remove to a wire cake rack.

To make the filling, beat together the ricotta, yoghurt,

honey and lemon and lime zest until smooth. Divide the mixture into three portions.

Remove the baking parchment from the base of the meringue layers. Place one meringue layer on a serving platter. Spread on, evenly, one of the lemon cheese filling portions. Place another meringue layer on top of this, then spread on the next portion of filling. Place the third layer of meringue on top and coat the top and sides of the cake with the remaining lemon cheese mixture.

Cover and refrigerate for 2 hours.

Place the water and sugar in a saucepan and bring to a rapid boil. Add the julienned lime zest and boil for 3–4 minutes, until the syrup becomes quite thick. (Do not allow it to colour.) Leave the mixture to cool.

Remove the cake from the refrigerator and sprinkle the top with the syrupy lime zest.

Serve small slices with fresh mint or fruit purée.

Serves 8 to 10

INGREDIENTS

BASE

4 egg whites

⅔ cup (155 g, 5 oz) caster (superfine) sugar

⅔ cup (100 g, 3½ oz) ground roasted almonds

⅓ cup (45 g, 1½ oz) cornflour (cornstarch)

1½ tablespoons icing (powdered) sugar

FILLING

500 g (16 oz) low-fat ricotta cheese

⅓ cup (90 mL, 3 fl oz) low-fat natural yoghurt

2 tablespoons honey

finely grated zest of 1 lemon

finely grated zest of 1 lime

DECORATION

¾ cup (185 mL, 6 fl oz) water

½ cup (125 g, 4 oz) sugar

zest of 3 limes, cut into julienne

fresh mint or fruit purée, for serving

Split Berry Bavarois

Stir the gelatine into the hot water and leave to soak.

Place the strawberry purée and the sugar in a small saucepan and slowly bring to a simmer. Remove from the heat and add the soaked gelatine. Stir well to combine.

Lightly brush 6 dariole moulds with oil and pour the strawberry mixture into the moulds. Refrigerate till set (about 1 hour).

Place the skim milk and the vanilla bean in a saucepan and bring to a rapid boil. Remove from the heat and leave to infuse for 10 minutes. Remove the bean and scrape the seeds into the milk.

Beat the eggs and sugar in a bowl until light and fluffy, then stir in the hot milk. Return the mixture to the saucepan and cook over a low heat, stirring constantly, until it has thickened enough to coat the back of a spoon. Do not allow the mixture to boil.

Dissolve the gelatine in the water. Stir the dissolved gelatine into the thickened liquid. When the gelatine has been incorporated, place the mixture over ice until it cools and thickens again. Quickly fold through the yoghurt.

Pour the mixture onto the set strawberry layer and refrigerate until the dessert has set firm (1–2 hours).

Unmould each bavarois onto a plate and serve with natural yoghurt, fresh berries and berry purée and a sprig of fresh mint.

Serves 6

1½ tablespoons powdered gelatine

¼ cup (60 mL, 2 fl oz) hot water

2 cups (500 mL, 16 fl oz) puréed strawberry pulp

1 tablespoon sugar

2 cups (500 mL, 16 fl oz) low-fat skim milk

1 vanilla bean

2 eggs

1 tablespoon sugar

1½ tablespoons powdered gelatine

¼ cup (60 mL, 2 fl oz) cold water

225 g (7 oz) low-fat plain natural yoghurt

DECORATION

low-fat plain natural yoghurt

fresh berries

berry purée

sprigs of fresh mint

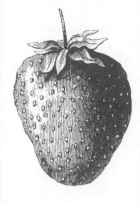

53

F
A
T

F
R
E
E

A
N
D

L
O
W

F
A
T

D
E
S
S
E
R
T
S

Angel Food Cake

Preheat the oven to 180°C (350°F).

Grease a 23 cm (9 in) springform cake tin lightly with butter. Place a circle of non-stick baking parchment on the base of the pan.

Sift the flours together.

Beat the egg whites, cream of tartar and lemon juice until stiff peaks form, then gradually beat in the caster sugar, a spoonful at a time. Continue beating until the sugar is dissolved.

Very gently fold through the flours and vanilla.

Pour the mixture into the prepared pan and bake for 45–50 minutes. The top should spring back when lightly touched.

Let the cake cool in the pan, then carefully remove it.

Serve the cake without decoration or garnishes for a sweet (but plain) snack, or serve lightly toasted slices with fresh fruit compôte over the top (or sandwich two slices with the fruit compôte).

Serves 8 to 10

INGREDIENTS

ANGEL FOOD CAKE

170 g (5½ oz) plain (all-purpose) flour

30 g (1 oz) cornflour (cornstarch)

8 egg whites

¼ level teaspoon cream of tartar

3 drops lemon juice

310 g (10 oz) caster (superfine) sugar

3 teaspoons vanilla extract

fresh fruit compote, for serving

DRUNKEN PLUMS

4 cups (1 litre, 32 fl oz) weak tea

1 cinnamon stick (quill)

finely grated zest of 1 lemon

finely grated zest of 1 orange

2 cups (1.5 kg, 2½ lb) purple plums, washed, pitted and cut into half

1 lemon, cut in half and sliced thinly

1 cup (250 mL, 8 fl oz) gin

low-cholesterol ice cream or fresh fruits, for serving

Drunken Plums

In a large saucepan, place the tea, cinnamon stick, lemon and orange zest, plum halves and sliced lemon. Bring slowly to the boil over a gentle heat.

Simmer, covered, for 20 minutes, then remove from the heat and let stand until cool.

Carefully pack two 1 litre (32 fl oz) glass jars evenly with the plums.

Pour ½ cup of the gin into each jar, then top the jars up with the tea and lemon slices.

Store for 1–2 weeks in the refrigerator before serving.

Serve on their own, or with low cholesterol ice cream, or with fresh fruits.

Serves 6 to 8

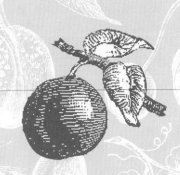

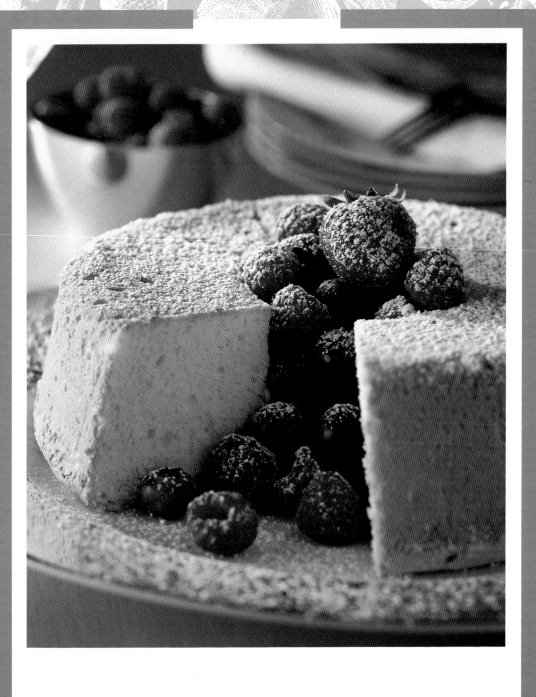

Angel Food Cake

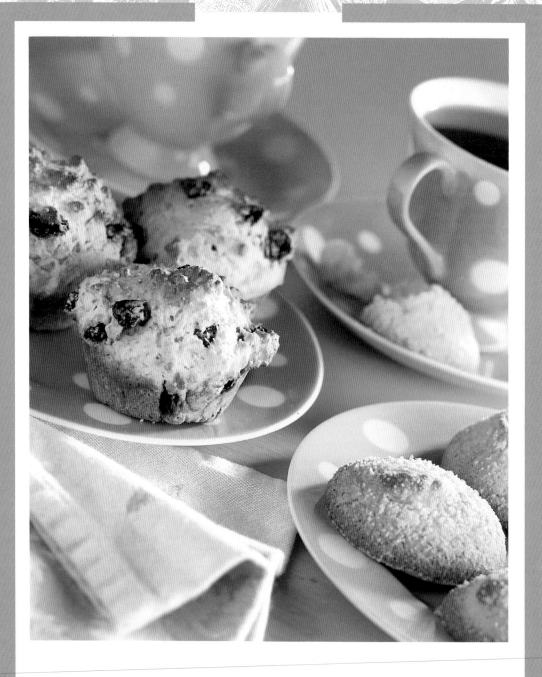

Wholemeal Lemon and Sultana Muffins with Orange Almandines

Orange Almandines

Preheat the oven to 160°C (325°F). Line 2 baking trays (sheets) with non-stick baking parchment.

Whisk the egg whites with ¼ cup of sugar until they form stiff peaks.

In a blender or food processor, grind the remaining cup of sugar, the almonds and orange zest.

Whisk the sugar and almond mixture into the egg whites.

Using a 1 cm (½ in) plain round nozzle fitted to a piping (pastry) bag, pipe 5 cm (2 in) fingers or 2 cm (1 in) discs of the mixture onto the prepared trays. Bake in the preheated oven until lightly golden brown, 12–15 minutes.

Leave on the tray to cool.

Makes 18 to 24

ORANGE ALMANDINES

3 egg whites

¼ cup (60 g, 2 oz) caster (superfine) sugar

1 cup (225 g, 7 oz) caster (superfine) sugar, extra

2 cups (250 g, 8 oz) ground almonds

finely grated zest of 1 orange

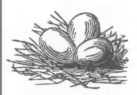

WHOLEMEAL LEMON AND SULTANA MUFFINS

1 cup (125 g, 4 oz) wholemeal (whole-wheat) plain flour

1 cup (125 g, 4 oz) plain (all-purpose) flour

4 teaspoons baking powder (soda)

½ teaspoon ground cloves

2 tablespoons sugar

60 g (2 oz) sultanas

zest and juice of 1 lemon

1 cup (250 mL, 8 fl oz) low-fat skim milk

1 egg white

Wholemeal Lemon and Sultana Muffins

Preheat the oven to 180°C (350°F). Place a paper patty case in each muffin space in a small 12-muffin tray.

Sift the flours, baking powder and cloves into a mixing bowl. Stir through the sugar. Add the sultanas, then the lemon juice and zest, milk and egg white.

Mix until just combined. Be careful not to overmix.

Spoon the mixture into 10 of the muffin cases, and bake in the preheated oven for 35–30 minutes.

Serve warm.

Makes 10

Crème de la Coeur

Blend the cheeses in a blender or food processor until any lumps are removed and they are of a smooth consistency.

Combine all ingredients in a bowl.

Line 4–6 small crème de la coeur moulds (heart-shaped moulds with small drainage holes in their bases) with muslin cloth (cheese cloth) or line one large mould (use a strainer or colander) with muslin cloth.

INGREDIENTS

1 cup (250 g, 8 oz)
low-fat ricotta cheese

2 cups (405 g, 13 oz)
low-fat cottage cheese

3 tablespoons
low-fat skim milk powder

⅓ cup (125 g, 4 oz) honey

¼ cup (30 g, 1 oz) walnuts,
chopped and roasted

½ cup (75 g, 2½ oz)
dried apricots, chopped

raspberry coulis, for serving

Fill the mould/s with the mixture. Weigh down the top/s of the mould/s to force out excess moisture, then refrigerate overnight.

Unmould directly onto the serving plate/s and serve with raspberry coulis.

Serves 4 to 6

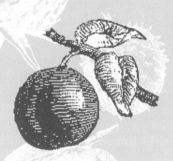

Snow Eggs

Whisk the egg whites until they form stiff peaks. Gradually add the sugar, still whisking.

Place the milk, sugar and vanilla bean in a saucepan and bring to the boil. Reduce the heat to a simmer. Place tablespoonfuls of the meringue in the simmering milk. Turn the meringues over and over until they are set firm, about 3–4 minutes.

Carefully remove the meringues. Serve them immediately, 'floating' on the citrus sauce.

Serves 4 to 6

SNOW EGGS

5 egg whites

225 g (7 oz) sugar

2 cups (500 mL, 16 fl oz) low-fat skim milk

1 vanilla bean

¼ cup (60 g, 2 oz) sugar

1 quantity of citrus sauce (see page 64)

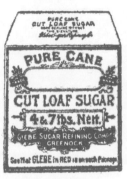

SWEET BREAD BUNS

1½ cups (185 g, 6 oz) plain (all-purpose) flour

½ cup (60 g, 2 oz) wholemeal (whole-wheat) plain flour

4 teaspoons baking powder (soda)

30 g (1 oz) sugar

½ teaspoon cinnamon

2 tablespoons currants

1 cup (250 mL, 8 fl oz) low-fat skim milk

skim milk, for brushing

Sweet Bread Buns

Preheat the oven to 200°C (400°F). Line a baking tray (sheet) with non-stick baking parchment.

Put all the dry ingredients in a bowl and make a well. Add the milk and mix until just combined. Do not overhandle the mixture.

Break into 10 even but rough pieces and place them on the baking tray. They will probably touch each other.

Brush the tops with skim milk and bake for 10–12 minutes.

Serve hot, warm or cold, buttered, with desserts, jam or koshav (see page 51).

Makes 10 buns

FAT FREE AND LOW FAT DESSERTS

Banana and Cinnamon Soufflé

Preheat the oven to 200°C (400°F).

Purée the banana with the lemon juice in a food processor or blender.

Whisk the egg whites until they form stiff peaks.

Fold the egg and banana mixtures together gently.

Divide the mixture among 6 lightly buttered individual soufflé dishes (ramekins) and bake for 15 minutes. Serve immediately.

INGREDIENTS

4 medium bananas

½ teaspoon lemon juice

4 egg whites

SAUCE

3 bananas

1 tablespoon lemon juice

2 tablespoons orange juice

½ teaspoon grated orange rind

4 tablespoons low-fat yoghurt or cottage cheese

To make the sauce, blend all the ingredients well in a blender or food processor.

Serves 6

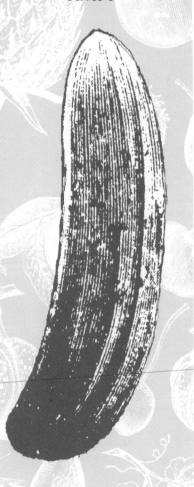

Apricot Whip

Mix the sugar with the stewed apricots in a large mixing bowl. Roughly chop the bread slices and mix these into the apricot mixture. Stir in the cinnamon.

Refrigerate the mixture until required (at least 20 minutes).

In a small bowl, dissolve the gelatine in the boiling water. Add the sugar to the dissolved gelatine mixture whilst it is still hot and then let the mixture cool slightly.

Add this mixture to the chilled evaporated milk and whisk at high speed until the mixture becomes thick and aerated.

INGREDIENTS

2 cups (500 mL, 16 fl oz) stewed apricots

30 g (1 oz) sugar

2 slices dried white bread (1–2 days old), crusts removed

1 teaspoon cinnamon

1½ teaspoons powdered gelatine

¼ cup (60 mL, 2 fl oz) boiling water

30 g (1 oz) sugar

¼ cup (60 mL, 2 fl oz) evaporated skim milk, well chilled

sponge fingers and fresh fruit, for serving

Fold this mixture through the apricot mixture and spoon immediately into parfait glasses.

Refrigerate the parfaits for 30–60 minutes, then serve with sponge fingers and fresh fruit.

This recipe would be delicious if made from a berry purée, such as raspberry, blackberry or strawberry. For these, though, use only 1½ cups of purée and chop 3–4 sprigs of fresh mint through the finished whip before pouring it into parfait glasses.

Serves 4 to 6

Gluhwein-marinated Citrus Salad

In a large saucepan, place all ingredients except the mandarin, orange and grapefruit segments.

Bring the mixture to the boil over a gentle heat, then let it simmer for 5 minutes.

Remove the simmered mixture from the heat and add the mandarin, orange and grapefruit segments. Leave the mixture to cool, then place it in the refrigerator for 24 hours.

Remove the mixture from the refrigerator and bring it to the boil again, over a low heat.

Scoop out the fruit segments and place them, with some of the lemon and orange zest, on a small plate for every person to help themselves.

INGREDIENTS

2 cups (500 ml, 16 fl oz) red wine

1 cup (250 mL, 8 fl oz) sauterne

90 g (3 oz) sugar

zest and juice of 2 lemons

zest of 1 orange

2 cinnamon sticks

4 cloves

5 mandarins, peeled and segmented and cleaned of fibrous pith

3 grapefruit, peeled and segmented and cleaned of fibrous pith

3 oranges, peeled and segmented and cleaned of fibrous pith

sprigs of fresh mint and low-fat natural yoghurt, for serving

Strain the remaining liquid and serve a small glass of this to each person.

Serve the fruit segments with a sprig of fresh mint and some low-fat natural yoghurt.

Serves 4 to 6

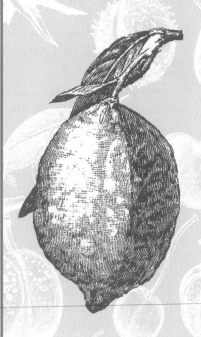

Pumpkin and Raspberry Brulées

Preheat the oven to 180°C (350°F).

Steam or boil the pumpkin until tender. Let the pumpkin cool then place it in a blender or food processor with the cottage cheese, eggs, honey and cinnamon and purée until smooth.

Place the mixture in a bowl and fold through the raspberries.

Pour the mixture into six soufflé ramekins and place them in a baking pan. Add water to the pan, to a depth of 6 mm (¼ in).

Bake the custards for 45 minutes, then remove them from the water bath and let them cool.

INGREDIENTS

2 cups (500 g, 16 oz) pumpkin

2 cups (500 g, 16 oz) low-fat cottage cheese

4 eggs

¼ cup (90 g, 3 oz) honey

¼ teaspoon cinnamon

1 cup (100 g, 3½ oz) fresh or frozen raspberries

100 g (3½ oz) sugar, for glazing

Refrigerate for 1 hour when cool and then sprinkle their tops with the sugar and glaze the tops of each under the grill or using a gas gun (torch).

Serves 6

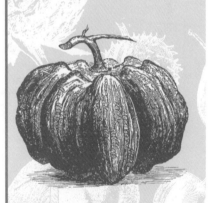

Citrus Sauce

Place the water, sugar, vanilla bean and lemon, orange and lime zests and lemon juice in a saucepan. Bring the mixture slowly to the boil and simmer it for 4–5 minutes.

Remove from the heat. Take out the vanilla pod, split it and scrape the seeds into the syrup mixture.

Let the liquid cool.

Place the cooled liquid, skim milk powder and honey in a food processor or blender and purée for 1–2 minutes.

INGREDIENTS

½ cup (125 mL, 4 fl oz) water

100 g (3½ oz) sugar

½ vanilla bean (pod)

finely grated zest of 1 lemon

finely grated zest of
1 orange

finely grated zest of 2 limes

3 teaspoons lemon juice

¾ cup skim milk powder

2 tablespoons honey

Place the sauce in the refrigerator for 1 hour, then serve with light desserts or with fresh fruit platters for a truly healthy alternative.

Serves 4

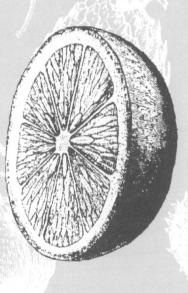

Raspberry Divinity

Cover the base of an oblong terrine or serving dish with the sponge fingers, laid flat, then sprinkle over the rum.

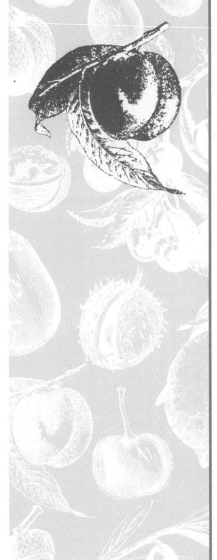

10 sponge fingers
(see page 110)

3 tablespoons rum

2⅓ cups (625 mL, 20 fl oz)
low-fat natural yoghurt

¾ cup (100 g, 3½ oz)
macadamia (Queensland)
nuts, lightly roasted and
chopped

60 g (2 oz) passionfruit pulp

1 cup (155 g, 5 oz)
fresh raspberries

4 tablespoons clear honey

passionfruit pulp, extra

raspberries, extra

fresh mint

icing (powdered) sugar,
for dusting

In a bowl, combine the yoghurt, macadamia nuts, passionfruit pulp, raspberries and honey.

Spread the yoghurt mixture evenly over the top of the sponge fingers. Refrigerate the dish for 2 hours before serving.

To serve, sprinkle the top with extra passionfruit pulp, fresh raspberries and some fresh mint, then dust lightly with icing sugar.

Serves 4 to 6

Apple, Raspberry and Apricot Puddings

Preheat the oven to 180°C (350°F). Very lightly oil six soufflé ramekins and place a small disc of non-stick baking parchment in the base of each.

Combine the grated apple, dried apricots and raspberries in a bowl.

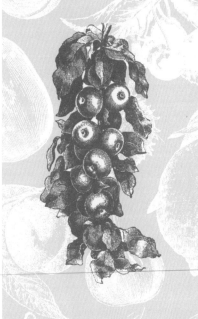

INGREDIENTS

1 medium apple, cored and grated

½ cup (90 g, 3 oz) dried apricots

1 cup (155 g, 5 oz) fresh raspberries

30 g (1 oz) skim milk powder

¼ cup (60 mL, 2 fl oz) orange juice

1 egg

2 teaspoons lemon juice

¼ teaspoon cinnamon

1 tablespoon golden syrup (light treacle)

30 g (1 oz) sugar

3 slices low-fat bread, broken into small pieces

icing (powdered) sugar, for dusting

In a separate bowl, lightly whisk the skim milk powder, orange juice, egg, lemon juice, cinnamon, golden syrup and sugar.

Pour the liquid over the fruits, add the broken bread crumbs and fold all together.

Fill the ramekins with the mixture and place them on a baking tray (sheet).

Bake in the preheated oven for 35–40 minutes.

Serve warm or cold, lightly dusted with icing sugar.

Serves 6

Light Tropical Roll

Preheat the oven to 180°C (350°F). Line the base of a 30 x 25 x 3 cm (12 x 10 x 1 in) baking tray (jelly roll pan) with non-stick baking parchment.

Place the eggs and sugar in a large bowl and whisk until light and fluffy.

Sift the flour and spices into a separate bowl.

In a third bowl whisk the egg whites until stiff peaks form. Still whisking, gradually add the golden syrup. Continue whisking until all is incorporated.

Fold the flour through the egg yolk mixture and then fold through the egg whites.

Spread the mixture evenly in the prepared tray.

Bake in the preheated oven for 20–25 minutes.

INGREDIENTS

4 eggs

½ cup (125 g, 4 oz) sugar

½ cup (60 g, 2 oz) plain (all-purpose) flour

1 teaspoon ground cinnamon

1 teaspoon mixed spice (five spice)

4 egg whites

1 tablespoon golden syrup (light treacle)

FILLING

250 g (8 oz) low-fat ricotta cheese

30 g (1 oz) dried apricots, finely chopped

30 g (1 oz) glacé pineapple, finely chopped

icing (powdered) sugar, for dusting

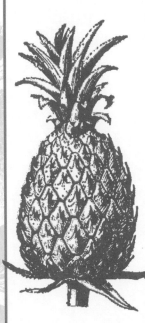

Turn out the sponge sheet onto a sheet of non-stick baking parchment lightly sprinkled with sugar.

Place the sponge sheet with its longer sides away from you. Roll up the sponge towards yourself, with the paper still enclosed. Leave the rolled-up sponge to cool (it will keep its shape).

To make the filling, beat the cheese until creamy, then stir through the chopped apricots and pineapple.

Unroll the cold sponge roll and spread it evenly with the filling. Reroll the sponge, but this time remove the paper as the roll is curled forward.

Dust lightly with icing sugar and refrigerate until served.

Serves 6 to 8

Spiced Coffee Bread

Line a 30 x 28 x 3 cm (12 x 11 x 1 in) baking tray (jelly roll pan) with non-stick baking parchment.

Place the water, sugar and honey in a large saucepan and slowly bring to the boil, stirring continuously. Leave to cool.

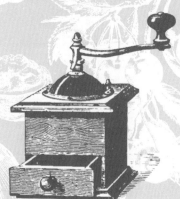

INGREDIENTS

1 cup (250 mL, 8 fl oz) water

¾ cup (185 g, 6 oz) sugar

¾ cup (280 g, 9 oz) honey

2½ cups (310 g, 10 oz) rye flour

2½ cups (310 g, 10 oz) plain (all-purpose) flour

1 teaspoon mixed spice (five spice)

½ teaspoon cinnamon

2 teaspoons baking powder (soda)

2 tablespoons mixed (candied) peel

4 egg yolks

Sift the flours, spices and baking powder into a large bowl.

Pour in the honey mixture, then the mixed peel and egg yolks and stir until all is combined.

Pour the mixture into the lined pan and bake in the preheated oven for 60–70 minutes.

Cool the slice in the tin and then cut very thin slices and serve with coffee or on a cheese board.

Makes 12 to 18 slices

Josef Cake

Preheat the oven to 180°C (350°F). Line the base of a 23 cm (9 in) springform cake tin with non-stick baking parchment.

Sift the flour, cornflour and cinnamon and leave to one side.

In a bowl, whisk the egg yolks, icing sugar and lemon zest until light and fluffy.

Place the egg whites in a separate bowl and whisk until they form stiff peaks. Add the icing sugar, a spoonful at a time. Continue whisking until the sugar is dissolved and incorporated.

Fold the egg whites, the flour mixture and the mixed peel into the egg yolk mixture.

Pour the batter into the prepared tin and bake until it springs back when touched lightly on top, 40–45 minutes.

INGREDIENTS

¾ cup (90 g, 3 oz) plain (all-purpose) flour

¾ cup (90 g, 3 oz) cornflour (cornstarch)

½ teaspoon cinnamon

6 egg yolks

⅔ cup (125 g, 4 oz) icing (powdered) sugar

zest of 1 lemon

6 egg whites

⅔ cup (125 g, 4 oz) icing (powdered) sugar, extra

30 g (1 oz) mixed (candied) peel

½ cup (125 g, 4 oz) low-fat natural yoghurt, for serving

fresh fruit, for serving

Dust lightly with icing sugar and serve (warm or cold) in small slices with the natural yoghurt and fresh fruit.

Serves 8 to 10

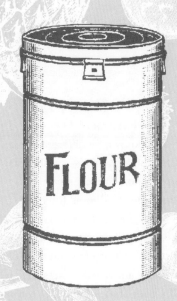

GLUTEN-FREE DESSERTS

The intolerance to gluten-based products is known by different names in different parts of the world — coeliac disease, coeliac sprue, non-tropical sprue and gluten intolerance — but in the main, those names refer to the same complaint.

Coeliacs are sensitive to gluten (the protein portion of wheat, rye, oats, barley, triticale and some millets). Gluten damages the cells of their small bowel (intestine).

This causes the loss of the tiny villi (small finger-like projections on the lining of the bowel). The cells of the villi (in a healthy intestine) help break down and absorb food nutrients. The coeliac sufferer, therefore, who has fewer of these cells and has some damaged cells as well, will also suffer deficiencies in vitamins, iron, folic acid and calcium because of the poor absorption of nutrients into the body.

The exact reason for this sensitivity and reaction to gluten is unknown. It may be an enzyme deficiency, causing the unnatural breakdown of gluten and the accumulation of a toxic portion, or it may be an abnormal immune reaction to the 'foreign' (non-human) gluten. It is also thought that coeliac disease can be triggered by stress, emotional and physical hardship and/or pregnancy.

Whilst coeliac disease has been diagnosed most often in young infants and children until recently, a high proportion of new diagnoses are of adults. The disease is thought to be hereditary and coeliacs remain sensitive throughout their lives. Some coeliacs suffer with small ailments for many years, even until adulthood, before they are correctly diagnosed. Coeliacs are never cured, but when gluten is removed from their diets, they return to normal lives.

Coeliac disease rates vary amongst countries and races. There are many thousands of sufferers in Australia, the USA and the United Kingdom and whilst other countries do have occurrences, the numbers of occurrences are unknown.

Common symptoms of sufferers are weight loss (and the inability to gain weight in younger children), tiredness, difficulties with conception, osteoporosis and diarrhoea. However, symptoms vary, and each case is different in many ways. Though the disease cannot be cured, it can be controlled by careful adherence to the appropriate diet.

Coeliac disease can be life-threatening so coeliacs need to know how to check food labels: sprays on common cereals can contain malt, which contains gluten, and some cornflours and custard powders also contain the protein. Wheat or gluten may also appear under other names — wheat flour, wheat starch, wheat bran, wheat meal, breadcrumbs, corn flour, baking flour, cake flour, pasta, spaghetti, all-purpose flour and self-raising (rising) flour — so a careful eye must be used when purchasing.

As most coeliacs are aware, even though it is easy enough to find foods without gluten, the continued eating of only these foods can lead to a deficiency in fibre, vitamin B1 and other complex carbohydrates. So a coeliac diet must compensate for this, not merely eliminate all gluten.

As with all allergies or intolerances, the advice of a dietitian and medical practitioner should be sought after diagnosis.

The desserts in this chapter offer coeliacs a new way to enjoy foods which are otherwise denied them.

Remember, though, that until a cure is found, careful selection of foods and a balanced diet will always be required.

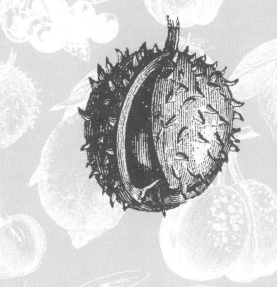

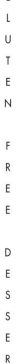

Japonaise Torte

The original recipe for this delight was made without flour, so it is a true winner for coeliacs.

Preheat the oven to 180°C (350°F). Line two baking sheets (trays) with non-stick baking parchment and draw a 23 cm (9 in) circle on each.

Whisk the egg whites until they form stiff peaks, then gradually add the sugar, a spoonful at a time. Beat at top speed on the mixer for 5 minutes, until the sugar is completely dissolved.

In another bowl, mix the almonds, cornflour and icing sugar. Very gently fold in the beaten egg whites (use a spatula).

Spoon half the mixture carefully onto each marked circle, spreading it to fill the disc, but staying inside the marked outline.

Bake for 30 minutes, then remove the meringue discs from the trays and let them cool (leave them on the parchment).

INGREDIENTS

BASE

4 egg whites

⅔ cup (155 g, 5 oz) caster (superfine) sugar

⅔ cup (100 g, 3½ oz) roasted almonds, ground

⅓ cup (45 g, 1½ oz) cornflour (maize) (cornstarch)

1½ tablespoons icing (powdered) sugar

BUTTERCREAM

155 g (5 oz) sugar

90 mL (3 fl oz) water

3 egg whites

250 g (8 oz) unsalted butter

¼ teaspoon ground cinnamon

2 cups flaked roasted almonds

icing (powdered) sugar, for dusting

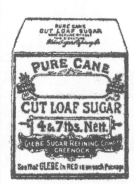

When the meringue discs are cool, remove the parchment. Spread one disc with buttercream, then top it with the second disc.

Cover the top and sides of the torte with buttercream, then press the flaked almonds onto the buttercream (top and sides) and dust the whole torte lightly with icing sugar.

Spread the buttercream on according to your own taste — if you use it all, it may be too rich for many people.

Chill for 1 hour, then serve.

TO MAKE THE BUTTERCREAM

Place the sugar and water in a saucepan and bring to the boil. Cook until the temperature reaches 115°C (240°F) on a sugar (candy) thermometer.

Whisk the egg whites until they form soft peaks, then beat in the hot syrup, a little at a time. When all the syrup has been added, continue beating until the mixture is cold.

In another bowl, beat the butter until it is light and creamy, then add the cinnamon. Fold this mixture into the cooled egg whites.

Serves 8 to 10

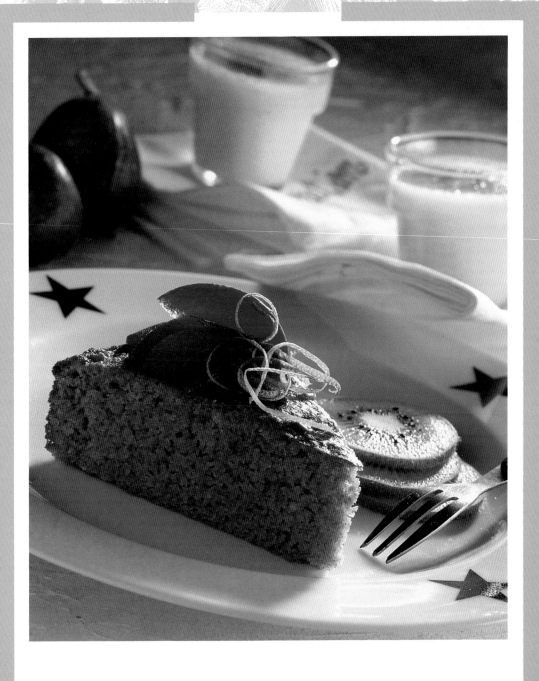

Cinnamon Almond Flan (front, page 80) and Lemon Curd Pots (page 81)

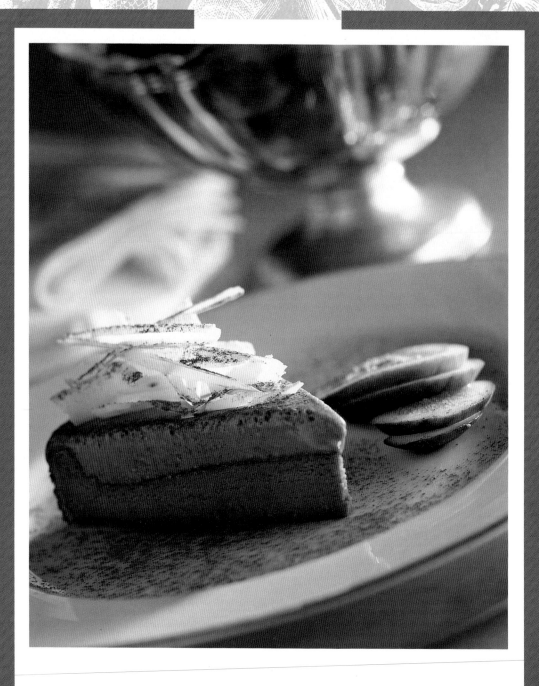

Chocolate Mousse Torte

Chocolate Mousse Torte

Preheat the oven to 180°C (350°F). Lightly grease a 20 cm (8 in) springform cake tin and place a disc of non-stick baking parchment on its base.

Beat the egg yolks and sugar until thick and almost white. Then gently beat in (by hand) the melted chocolate and melted butter.

In another bowl, whisk the egg whites until they form stiff peaks. Fold the egg whites into the chocolate mixture.

Pour three-quarters of the mixture into the prepared tin and bake for 45 minutes, or until the mixture has shrunk away from the sides slightly.

Let the cake cool in the tin (it will sink in the middle).

When the cake is cold, pour the reserved quarter of the mixture into the centre of the cake.

Refrigerate overnight.

Remove the cake carefully from the cake tin, dust lightly with cocoa and serve in slices with fresh berries.

Serves 8 to 10

CHOCOLATE MOUSSE TORTE

8 egg yolks

75 g (2½ oz) sugar

250 g (8 oz) dark (plain or semi-sweet) chocolate, melted

125 g (4 oz) unsalted butter, melted

8 egg whites

fresh berries, for serving

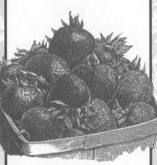

PAVLOVA

4 egg whites

¼ cup (60 g, 2 oz) icing (powdered) sugar

225 g (6 oz) sugar

3 tablespoons cornflour (maize) (cornstarch)

3 tablespoons unsweetened cocoa powder

1⅓ cups (310 mL, 10 fl oz) single (light, whipping) cream, freshly whipped

fresh fruit

Pavlova

Preheat the oven to 90°C (180°F). Line a baking tray (sheet) with non-stick baking parchment marked with a 20 cm (8 in) circle.

Whisk the egg whites until they form stiff peaks.

Combine the icing sugar and sugar and slowly add them, a spoonful at a time, to the egg whites. Keep whisking until all the sugar is dissolved. Carefully fold the cornflour and cocoa through.

Spread the mixture over the marked circle on the baking parchment. Place the baking tray in the oven and bake for 2 hours. Turn off the oven, but leave the pavlova in the oven to cool, preferably overnight.

When the pavlova is completely cold, peel off the baking parchment and place the pavlova on a serving dish.

Spread the pavlova with the whipped cream, then place a selection of fresh fruits on top.

Refrigerate until needed. Serve with a light berry sauce or coulis.

Serves 6 to 8

Fruit Cake

Preheat the oven to 180°C (350°F). Line a 24 x 12 x 8 cm (10 x 5 x 3 in) loaf tin with non-stick baking parchment.

Sift the flours, skim milk powder and baking powder together.

In a bowl, beat the eggs with the sugar and melted butter, then add this mixture to the dry ingredients to form a batter.

Stir the fruits through the batter thoroughly.

Pour the batter into the prepared loaf tin and bake for 45–50 minutes, or until a skewer inserted into the top comes out clean.

Cool in the pan (for about 1 hour) before removing. Serve in slices.

Makes 12 to 14 slices

INGREDIENTS

FRUIT CAKE

1 cup (155 g, 5 oz) rice flour

1 cup (125 g, 4 oz) potato flour

⅔ cup (45 g, 1½ oz) skim milk powder

2½ teaspoons baking powder (soda)

2 eggs

½ cup (125 g, 4 oz) caster (superfine) sugar

125 g (4 oz) unsalted butter, melted

¾ cup (125 g, 4 oz) sultanas

1 cup (125 g, 4 oz) chopped dates

1 cup (125 g, 4 oz) chopped dried apricots

1 cup (125 g, 4 oz) currants

TROPICAL ENGLISH RICE PUDDING

1 cup (225 g, 7 oz) raw short grain white rice

1 cup (250 mL, 8 fl oz) milk

1¼ cups (310 mL, 10 fl oz) water

90 g (3 oz) brown sugar (light)

¼ teaspoon ground cloves

2 teaspoons cornflour (maize) (cornstarch)

1 fresh mango, flesh cut into thin slices

Tropical English Rice Pudding

Cook the rice in a saucepan of boiling water for 10–12 minutes, until tender. Drain and set aside.

Combine the milk, water, brown sugar and cloves in a large saucepan. Bring to the boil, then stir in the cooked rice. Reduce the heat and simmer for 15 minutes.

Add the cornflour, blended with a little water, and stir until the rice boils again. Fold through the mango slices and serve warm.

Serves 6

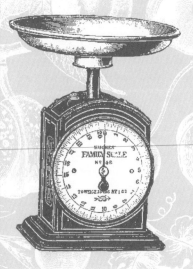

Baked Cheesecake

310 mL (10 fl oz) milk

30 g (1 oz) butter

250 g (8 oz) cream cheese

30 g (1 oz) sugar

125 mL (4 fl oz) milk, extra

60 g (2 oz) custard powder (gluten-free)

100 g (3½ oz) sultanas, soaked in hot water for 24 hours and drained

6 egg whites

100 g (3½ oz) sugar, extra

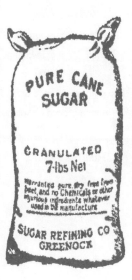

Preheat the oven to 180°C (350°F). Lightly grease a 20 cm (8 in) springform cake tin and place a sheet of non-stick baking parchment on its base.

Place the milk, butter, cream cheese and sugar in a saucepan and bring slowly to the boil. Whisk gently, until the cream cheese has broken down and the mixture is smooth, as the mixture is heating.

In a bowl, quickly blend the extra milk and custard powder into a paste. Beat this into the mixture as it heats.

Boil the mixture until it thickens, then remove from the heat and let it cool slightly. Fold through the sultanas.

Beat the egg whites until they form stiff peaks, then gradually whisk in the sugar, a spoonful at a time, until all is dissolved and incorporated.

Fold the egg whites into the cream cheese mixture.

Pour the mixture into the prepared tin.

Bake for 45–50 minutes, or until the cheesecake is golden brown on top and firm to the touch.

Let the cheesecake cool in the cake tin. It will sink considerably. When it is cool (after about 1 hour), run a knife around the outside edge of the cheesecake to loosen it from the tin.

Serve the cheesecake warm or cold.

Serves 8 to 10

GLUTEN FREE DESSERTS

Moist Almond Torte

Preheat the oven to 180°C (350°F). Lightly grease a 23 cm (9 in) springform cake tin with butter.

Place a handful of desiccated coconut in the tin and swirl it around so that it will cover (and stick to) the base and sides. Shake out the excess lightly.

Combine the almonds, coconut, sugar and butter, then add the lightly beaten eggs.

Pour the mixture into the tin and bake for 45 minutes. Let the cake cool a little in the tin, then invert it carefully onto a flat plate.

To Make the Buttercream

Place the sugar and water in a saucepan and bring to the boil. Cook until the temperature reaches 115°C (240°F) on a sugar (candy) thermometer.

Beat the egg whites until they form soft peaks, then beat in the hot syrup, a little at a time. When all the syrup has been added, continue beating until the mixture is cold.

Ingredients

185 g (6 oz)
ground (minced) almonds

60 g (2 oz) desiccated
(shredded) coconut

1 cup (250 g, 8 oz) sugar

225 g (7 oz)
unsalted butter, melted

4 eggs, lightly beaten

zest of 1 orange,
finely grated

zest of 1 orange and
1 lemon, for decorating

Buttercream

185 g (6 oz) sugar

100 mL (3½ fl oz) water

4 egg whites

250 g (8 oz) unsalted butter

¼ teaspoon ground cinnamon

Almond Praline

250 g (8 oz)
caster (superfine) sugar

250 g (8 oz) flaked almonds

orange and lemon zest,
for decoration

In another bowl, beat the butter until it is light and creamy, then add the cinnamon. Fold into the cooled egg white mixture.

Spread buttercream on top and around the sides of the torte. Do not spread it on too thickly. Leftover buttercream will keep for 4–5 days in an airtight container in the refrigerator.

To Make the Almond Praline

Heat an empty heavy-based saucepan over a medium heat. Slowly sprinkle some of the sugar into the pan. Let it melt before stirring in more. Keep adding the sugar until all is added and all is molten. Continue stirring until the sugar turns a light golden caramelised colour.

Stir in the almonds. Make sure they are all covered with caramel.

Pour the mixture onto a large sheet of non-stick baking parchment and spread it out gently, using a wooden spoon.

Place a second sheet of non-stick baking parchment on top of the praline. Use a rolling pin to roll the praline, while it is still hot, to a very fine thickness.

Leave the praline until it is cold and hard, then peel off the sheets of paper and break the praline into large pieces.

To Assemble the Cake

When the cake is completely cooled, spread the top and sides evenly with the buttercream.

Place some of the praline pieces around the sides of the cake. Crush the remainder of the praline and sprinkle into the centre of the cake with some orange and lemon zest.

Refrigerate for 2 hours then serve. This cake should be eaten within 48 hours of being made.

Serves 8 to 10

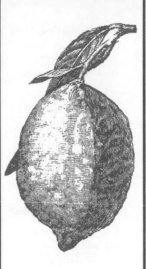

BERRY SOUFFLÉ

1½ cups (405 g, 13 oz)
raspberry purée

2 tablespoons sugar

4 egg whites

¼ teaspoon lemon juice

1 tablespoon sugar, extra

Berry Soufflé

From the chef's point of view, this is one of the lightest and most gratifying recipes to make. It is a light end to a heavy meal or just a nice flavour sensation for a light meal.

Preheat the oven to 200°C (400°F).

Place the raspberries and the sugar in a blender or food processor and reduce to a pulp.

Whisk the egg whites, lemon juice and sugar until they are stiff and fluffy.

Gently fold the egg whites through the raspberry pulp.

Pour the mixture into four lightly greased and sugared soufflé ramekins.

Place in the preheated oven and cook for 12–15 minutes, or until golden brown and well risen.

Serve immediately with some raspberry purée or chocolate sauce and whipped cream.

Serves 4

Cinnamon Almond Flan

Preheat the oven to 180°C (350°F). Lightly grease a 20 cm (8 in) deep quiche dish (pie dish).

In a bowl, whisk the eggs lightly.

Add the sugar, cream and milk and whisk lightly to incorporate all ingredients.

Stir in the cinnamon, ground almonds and baking powder.

Pour the mixture into the greased dish and bake for 40–45 minutes, or until firm to the touch.

Remove the flan from the oven, let it cool, then dust it with icing sugar.

Serve with fresh cream, fresh fruit or a berry sauce.

Serves 8 to 10

INGREDIENTS

CINNAMON ALMOND FLAN

3 eggs

¾ cup (185 g, 6 oz) sugar

⅔ cup (155 mL, 5 fl oz) single (light, whipping) cream

⅔ cup (155 mL, 5 fl oz) milk

3 teaspoons ground cinnamon

2 cups (225 g, 7 oz) ground almonds

1 tablespoon baking powder (soda)

icing (powdered) sugar, for dusting

cream (single or double), fresh fruit or berry sauce, for serving

CORNFLOUR SPONGE

4 eggs

¾ cup (185 g, 6 oz) caster (superfine) sugar

½ cup (60 g, 2 oz) custard powder (gluten-free)

½ cup (60 g, 2 oz) cornflour (maize) (cornstarch)

1 teaspoon cream of tartar

½ teaspoon bicarbonate of soda

Cornflour Sponge

Preheat the oven to 180°C (350°F). Lightly grease 2 deep sandwich sponge tins (15 cm/6 in diameter) and line the bases with non-stick baking parchment.

In a large bowl, whisk the eggs and sugar until thick and fluffy.

Sift the custard powder, cornflour, cream of tartar and bicarbonate of soda twice, then fold them through the egg mixture.

Spread the mixture into the 2 sponge tins and bake for 20–25 minutes, or until top springs back when touched.

These sponges have several uses: for the base of richer cake creations; sandwiched together with jam (jelly) and cream for an afternoon tea snack; sliced and used for zuccotta; bases of ice cream bombes; or wherever sponge or cake crumbs are required in other recipes.

Serves 6 to 8

Lemon Curd Pots

Preheat the oven to 180°C (350°F).

Lightly whisk the eggs in a stainless steel bowl. Stir through the sugar, then the lemon juice and zest. Chop the butter into small pieces and add it to the mixture.

Place the bowl over a bain-marie or saucepan of simmering water and whisk until the butter has melted. Keep whisking lightly until the mixture thickens and coats the back of a spoon.

Pour the mixture into 4 to 6 small soufflé ramekins and bake until the tops are golden brown, about 15–20 minutes.

Let the pots cool in the refrigerator for 3 hours, then dust lightly with icing sugar and serve each with a fresh strawberry.

Variation
Store your lemon curd in a jar in the refrigerator, then spread it cold onto a sponge, top with whipped cream and serve for morning or afternoon tea.

Serves 4 to 6

LEMON CURD POTS
3 eggs
zest and juice of 2 lemons
225 g (7 oz) sugar
155 g (5 oz) unsalted butter
icing (powdered) sugar, for dusting
fresh strawberries, for serving

RASPBERRY POLENTA CREAM
4 tablespoons polenta (cornmeal)
2 cups (500 mL, 16 fl oz) milk
2 tablespoons clear honey
2⅔ cups (700 g, 22 oz) fresh low-fat ricotta cheese
½ cup (125 g, 4 oz) raspberry jam
2 punnets (500 g, 16 oz) fresh or frozen raspberries

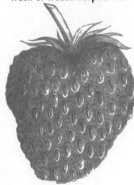

Raspberry Polenta Cream

Blend the polenta with ⅓ cup of the milk to form a paste.

Place the remaining milk in a saucepan and bring slowly to the simmer.

Add the polenta and stir, over the heat, until the mixture boils and thickens. Cook for 1 minute, then remove from the heat. Stir in the honey. Let the mixture cool.

In a blender or food processor, whip the ricotta, then stir in the jam and the cooled polenta mixture. Finally, fold the berries through, leaving some for decoration.

Pour the mixture into six parfait glasses and top with the remaining berries. Dust lightly with nutmeg or cinnamon sugar.

Serve well chilled.

Serves 6

Coconut Macaroons

Preheat the oven to 180°C (350°F). Line a baking tray (sheet) with non-stick baking parchment.

In a large saucepan, mix the coconut and sugar with a wooden spoon. Add the egg white and lemon juice and zest and stir to a moistened paste.

Place the saucepan over a low heat and stir continuously until the mixture reaches 40°C (104°F) on a sugar (candy) thermometer.

Remove the pan from the heat and continue stirring until the mixture cools.

Place the mixture in a piping (pastry) bag which has been fitted with a 1.5 cm (¾ in) star piping nozzle (tube).

Pipe small rosette shapes onto the baking sheet and bake for 10–15 minutes, or until the macaroons are golden brown. Cool on the baking tray, then store in an airtight container.

Makes 12 to 18

INGREDIENTS

COCONUT MACAROONS

3⅓ cups (310 g, 10 oz) desiccated (shredded) coconut

2 cups (500 g, 16 oz) sugar

225 mL (7 fl oz) egg white

juice and zest of 1 lemon

ORANGE CHOCOLATE MUFFINS

⅓ cup (60 g, 2 oz) potato flour

¼ cup (45 g, 1½oz) rice flour

3 teaspoons baking powder (soda)

½ cup (125 g, 4 oz) polenta (cornmeal)

30 g (1 oz) sugar

½ cup (125 mL, 4 fl oz) milk

1 egg, lightly beaten

⅓ cup (60 g, 2 oz) dark (plain or semi-sweet) chocolate, finely chopped

1½ cups (405 g, 13 oz) fresh orange segments

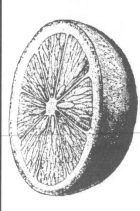

Orange Chocolate Muffins

Preheat the oven to 180°C (350°F). Lightly grease (or line with paper cases) a 10–12 cup muffin pan.

Sift the potato flour, rice flour and baking powder into a large bowl. Add the polenta and sugar and mix with a spoon.

Fold through the milk, egg, chocolate and orange segments. When all ingredients are moistened, pour the mixture into ten of the twelve muffin pans.

Bake for 30 minutes, or until golden.

Let the muffins cool in the pan for 2–3 minutes before carefully removing them. Serve warm or cold.

Serves 10

Luscious Coconut Cream Cake

Place the coconut cream, sugar and rum in a saucepan and bring to the boil.

Pour this liquid over the coconut and leave it to soak for 1 hour.

Pour the milk into a saucepan and bring to the boil.

In a bowl, combine the cornflour with the egg yolks, then pour in the hot milk, beating all the time.

Return the mixture to the saucepan and cook for 2 minutes, stirring continuously. Take this custard mixture off the heat, but keep it warm.

Whisk the egg whites until they form stiff peaks, then gradually add the sugar, a spoonful at a time, beating well until it is all incorporated and dissolved.

Fold the egg whites into the warm custard and then fold in the coconut mixture.

Cut the two sponges in half horizontally.

Spread one layer with some of the coconut mixture, place another layer of sponge on top, then top this with more of the mixture. Continue in this fashion with the next two layers of sponge, reserving a little of the coconut mixture to spread on the sides and top of the cake.

Press the toasted shredded coconut into the sides and on top, then dust the cake lightly with icing sugar and refrigerate for 2–3 hours before serving.

Serves 8 to 10

INGREDIENTS

2 cornflour (maize) (cornstarch) sponges (see page 80)

100 mL (3½ fl oz) coconut cream

1 cup (250 g, 8 oz) sugar

¼ cup (60 mL, 2 fl oz) rum

3⅓ cups (310 g, 10 oz) desiccated (shredded) coconut

100 mL (3½ fl oz) milk

3 tablespoons cornflour (maize) (cornstarch)

3 egg yolks

2 cups (500 mL, 16 fl oz) milk, extra

3 egg whites

¼ cup (60 g, 2 oz) sugar, extra

toasted shredded coconut, for decorating

icing (powdered) sugar, for decorating

Apple Upside-down Cake

Preheat the oven to 180°C (350°F). Lightly grease a 20 cm (8 in) springform cake tin and line its base with non-stick baking parchment.

Sift together the rice flour, potato flour and baking powder.

Combine the apple, sugar and cinnamon in a bowl. Spread this mixture evenly over the base of the tin.

In another bowl, cream the butter and sugar until smooth and creamy. Fold in the sifted dry ingredients and milk alternately. Pour the batter into the prepared cake tin, on top of the apple mixture.

Bake for 30–40 minutes. Let the cake cool, then turn it out, upside down, onto a plate. Remove the parchment paper and serve.

Serves 8 to 10

INGREDIENTS

APPLE UPSIDE-DOWN CAKE

½ cup (60 g, 2 oz) rice flour

½ cup (60 g, 2 oz) potato flour

2 teaspoons baking powder (soda)

1½ cups (225 g, 7 oz) stewed apple, well drained

2 tablespoons sugar

2 teaspoons cinnamon

4 tablespoons unsalted butter

¼ cup (60 g, 2 oz) sugar

1 egg

⅓ cup (90 mL, 3 fl oz) milk

CITRUS CRUMBLE

2 mandarins

3 oranges

2 pink grapefruit

pulp of 4 fresh passionfruit

¼ cup (60 g, 2 oz) apricot jam

4 tablespoons flaked almonds

4 tablespoons rice flour

2 tablespoons brown sugar (light)

4 tablespoons milk powder

125 g (4 oz) unsalted butter, melted

Citrus Crumble

Preheat the oven to 180°C (350°F).

Peel the mandarins, oranges and grapefruit and remove the pith. Cut the mandarins, oranges and grapefruit into segments and place them in the base of a 20 cm (8 in) quiche dish (pie dish).

Place the passionfruit pulp and the apricot jam in a saucepan and warm lightly over a low heat. Pour this mixture evenly over the mandarin, orange and grapefruit segments.

In a separate bowl, mix the remaining ingredients. When all are combined, sprinkle over the top of the fruit.

Bake for 25 minutes and serve warm.

Serves 4

Flourless Chocolate Cake

Since time began, or at least since the invention of block chocolate, I think there has always been a flourless chocolate cake.
This is yet another in the series, and a personal favourite for me.

Preheat the oven to 180°C (350°F). Line a 20 cm (8 in) springform cake tin with non-stick baking parchment.

Place the egg yolks in a bowl with the sugar and whisk until light and fluffy. In a separate bowl, whisk the egg whites until they form stiff peaks.

Fold the chocolate and sour cream into the egg yolk mixture, add the ground almonds, then gently fold in the egg whites.

6 eggs, separated

225 g (7 oz) sugar

500 g (1 lb) dark (plain or semi-sweet) chocolate, melted

½ cup (125 mL, 4 fl oz) sour cream

½ cup (60 g, 2 oz) ground almonds

marinated berries or double (heavy, thickened) cream, for serving

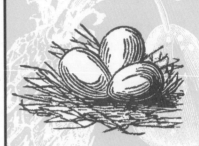

Pour the mixture into the tin and bake for 1 hour, or until a skewer inserted into the middle of the cake comes out clean. Remove from the oven and let the cake cool in the tin.

Serve the cake in slices, with marinated berries or thick cream.

Serves 8 to 10

Raspberry Cheesecake

Preheat the oven to 180°C (350°F). Lightly oil and line a 20 cm (8 in) springform cake tin with non-stick baking parchment.

BASE

Mix together the crushed cornflakes, coconut, cinnamon and melted butter. Press this mixture into the base of the tin. Chill.

FILLING

Sift the flour and baking powder together.

In a blender or food processor, blend the flour and baking powder, cream cheese, caster sugar and orange juice and zest until smooth.

Beat the egg whites until they form stiff peaks, then fold them into the mixture. Pour the mixture on top of the base. Bake for 1 hour, then leave to cool. Turn the cheesecake out gently onto a wire rack.

INGREDIENTS

BASE

½ cup (90 g, 3 oz) cornflakes (malt-free), crushed

¼ cup (30 g, 1 oz) desiccated (shredded) coconut, toasted

¼ teaspoon cinnamon

3 tablespoons melted butter

FILLING

½ cup (90 g, 3 oz) rice flour

2 teaspoons baking powder (soda)

1½ cups (375 g, 12 oz) cream cheese

½ cup (125 g, 4 oz) caster (superfine) sugar

juice and finely grated zest of 1 orange

4 egg whites

TOPPING

¼ teaspoon powdered gelatine

a little water

500 g (1 lb) fresh raspberries

½ cup (125 mL, 4 fl oz) orange juice

6 teaspoons sugar

TOPPING

Soften the gelatine in a little water.

Arrange the best-looking raspberries on top of the cheesecake. Place the rest in a saucepan with the orange juice, bring to the boil and boil for 8–10 minutes. Mash the berries into the liquid to extract as much flavour and colour as possible. Strain the liquid, then pass it through a sieve to remove the seeds.

Return the juice to the saucepan, add the sugar and bring to the boil again, stirring to make sure the sugar has dissolved. Add the softened gelatine and stir until it has dissolved. Remove the saucepan from the heat and let the mixture cool until it is just beginning to set.

Cover the cheesecake with raspberry glaze and chill overnight before serving.

Serves 12

Creamy Blackberry Tart

BASE

Mix together the crushed cornflakes, coconut, cinnamon and butter. Press into the base of a 20 cm (8 in) springform cake tin. Chill while you prepare the filling.

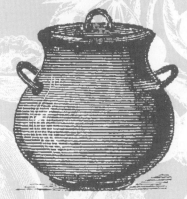

FILLING

Cream the butter and sugar together until light and fluffy.

Add the eggs, one at a time, and continue beating until all is combined and the mixture is light.

BASE

½ cup (90 g, 3 oz) cornflakes (malt-free), crushed

¼ cup (30 g, 1 oz) desiccated (shredded) coconut, toasted

60 g (2 oz) melted butter

¼ teaspoon cinnamon

FILLING

155 g (5 oz) unsalted butter

⅔ cup (155 g, 5 oz) caster (superfine) sugar

2 eggs

125 g (4 oz) good quality white chocolate, melted

½ teaspoon ground cinnamon

1 punnet (225 g, 7 oz) blackberries

DECORATIONS

1 punnet (225 g, 7 oz) blackberries

white chocolate curls

Add the melted chocolate to the butter mixture along with the cinnamon. When combined, carefully fold the blackberries through. Try not to damage the fruit.

Spoon the mixture onto the chilled base and press it flat with a spatula.

Press fresh blackberries onto the top and decorate with white chocolate curls.

Refrigerate for 3 hours before serving.

Serves 6 to 8

GLUTEN FREE DESSERTS

LACTOSE-FREE DESSERTS

Lactose is found in milk and dairy foods, and in manufactured foods containing milk. People who have a lactose intolerance are not able to break down this lactose. This causes them to experience some or all of a range of symptoms: belching, rumbling, feelings of fullness, bloating, wind pains, loose stools, diarrhoea. These symptoms can appear in a short time — within a few minutes — or several hours after eating. They are due to a lactase deficiency.

Lactase is an enzyme present in the cells of the surface of the small intestine. It breaks the lactose down into the simple sugars — glucose and galactose. After this, the sugars are easily absorbed into the body.

In a body deficient in lactase this reaction will not take place and the lactose will instead be digested by bacteria, leading to gas, diarrhoea and abdominal bloating or swelling. Many people have a genetic predisposition to lactose deficiency in adulthood, but it is usually not until early teenage years that it is diagnosed or even noticed. Whilst an intolerance to lactose is a cause of trauma to the body, it is almost a Catch 22 situation in that the more stress or trauma the person suffers, the greater the effects of the intolerance.

The symptoms of lactose intolerance often go untreated for many years due to wrong diagnosis or because only minor symptoms are seen and they are therefore ignored. Once diagnosed, talk to your dietitian to see how much or how little lactose you may have in your diet. Milk does play an important part in our body's growth and longevity and some components of milk, such as calcium, must be taken in tablet form if milk is not allowed at all. There are now some milks which have already been treated with lactase enzymes. This means a happier, safer and more wide-ranging culinary world is available for some with this complaint.

The second problem is an allergy to cows'

milk, more common in children but also seen in adults. This milk allergy is the more serious of the two types and can cause more violent and more widespread symptoms. The allergy is an immune response from the white blood cells to one or more milk proteins which, rather than protecting the body, may cause damage to the intestinal and bodily tissues, intestinal discomfort or more serious problems. Symptoms range from serious (vomiting excessively and suddenly, skin rashes, asthma and problems with breathing or circulation) to relatively minor (eczema and an increase or build-up of mucus).

Because there is such a range of symptoms, the allergy can be misdiagnosed for many years, especially in smaller children who cannot easily explain and describe their physical feelings and pains.

As with diabetes, I have had first-hand experience with people who have an intolerance to lactose. A close friend of mine has an allergy to cows' milk, and suffers severe asthma and mucus build-up after eating cheese, or yoghurt or too much milk, or after unwittingly eating other milk-containing foods.

If you are allergic to milk, you have to give up all dairy products. You may then need calcium supplements (which should include vitamin D). Your dietitian will advise you on what you can eat so that you can still lead a life which is safe and comfortable.

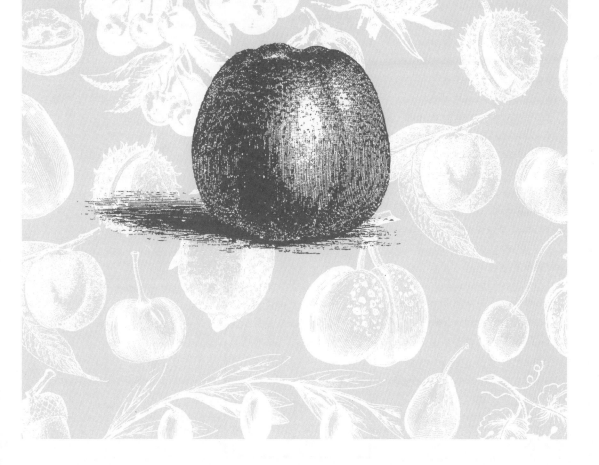

Glazed Spicy Fruit Loaf

Lightly grease (with oil) a 20 cm (8 in) springform cake tin.

Sift the flour and sugar with the cinnamon and cloves into a large mixing bowl.

In a separate bowl, mix the water and the yeast. Stir to dissolve the yeast. When the yeast is dissolved stir this liquid into the flour. Add the egg and the oil.

Work the mixture to a dough, then place it on a lightly floured surface. Knead well for 3–5 minutes.

Lightly knead in the currants, sultanas and peel. Return the dough to the bowl and cover with a damp cloth. Place the bowl in a warm position for 40 minutes, or until the dough has doubled in size.

Preheat the oven to 180°C (350°F).

Remove the risen dough from the bowl and knead the dough on a lightly floured surface to remove any air from it.

INGREDIENTS

3 cups (375 g, 12 oz) plain (all-purpose) flour

¼ cup (60 g, 2 oz) caster (superfine) sugar

½ teaspoon cinnamon

½ teaspoon ground cloves

1 cup (250 mL, 8 fl oz) water

30 g (1 oz) fresh compressed yeast

1 egg

3 tablespoons olive oil

½ cup (75 g, 2½ oz) currants

2 tablespoons sultanas (golden raisins)

30 g (1 oz) mixed (candied) peel

1 egg white, beaten

3 tablespoons raw sugar

1 teaspoon cinnamon

GLAZE

3 tablespoons water

1 tablespoon powdered gelatine

2 tablespoons sugar

Roll out the dough until it is 30 x 30 cm (12 x 12 in). Brush lightly with the beaten egg white, then sprinkle with the raw sugar and cinnamon.

Starting with the side furthest from you, roll the dough up tightly, like a Swiss roll. Cut the roll into 8 even portions and place these in the greased pan, cut ends upwards.

Place the pan in a warm area for a further 40 minutes, or until the dough has doubled in bulk, then bake for 30–35 minutes, or until golden brown.

TO MAKE THE GLAZE

Place all the ingredients in a saucepan and bring to the boil. Remove from the heat and brush over the cooked loaf pieces.

Serves 8

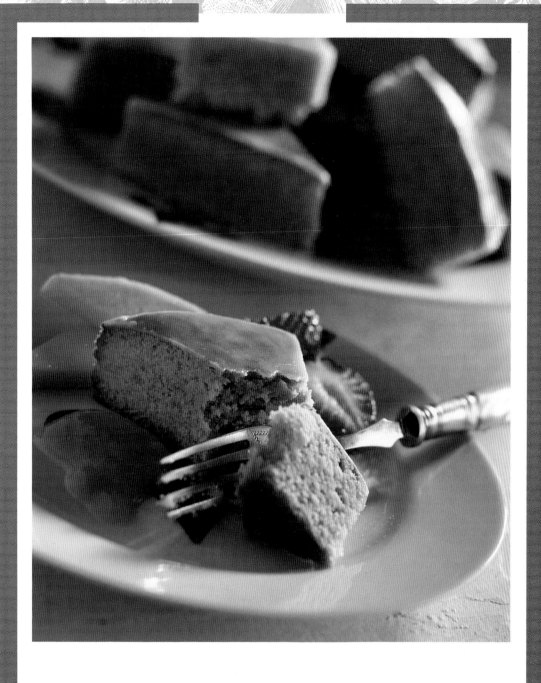

Honey Slice (page 98)

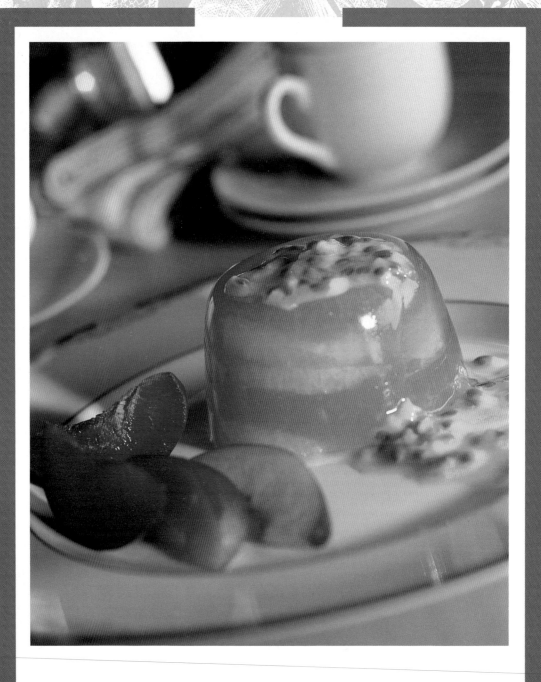

Sauterne and Citrus Jellies (page 97)

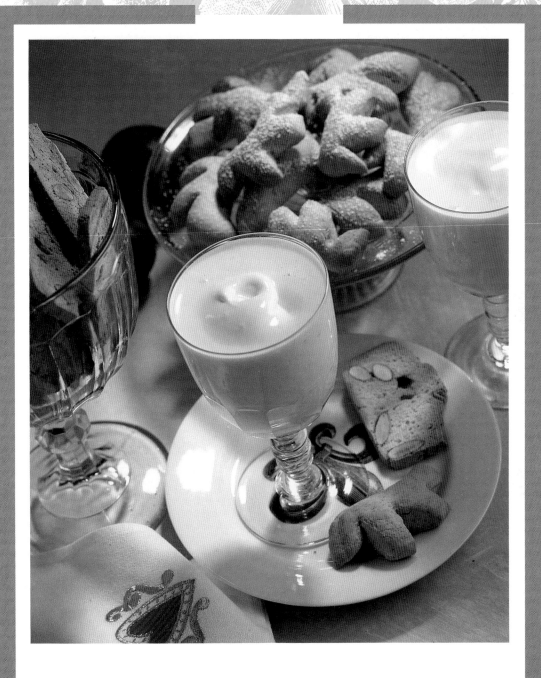

Almond Bread (left, page95), Mediterranean Clove Cookies (right, page 96) and Zabaglione (front, page 97)

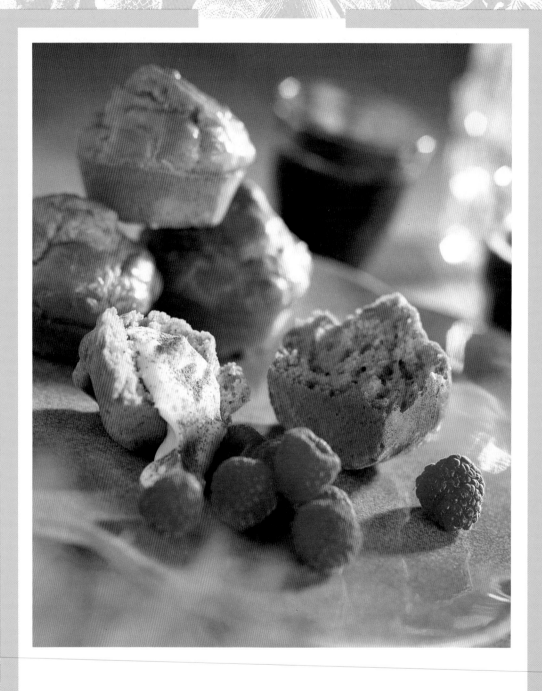

Sour Cream and Peanut Muffins (page 113)

Almond Bread

Preheat the oven to 180°C (350°F). Prepare a 24 x 7 x 5 cm (10 x 3 x 2 in) loaf tin by lightly greasing the sides and lining the base with non-stick baking parchment.

Sift the flour and cinnamon into a mixing bowl.

In a separate bowl, whisk the egg whites until they form stiff peaks. Gradually add the sugar, a spoonful at a time, beating well after each addition. Continue whisking until all the sugar has been incorporated and dissolved.

Carefully fold the flour and cinnamon and the nuts into the egg whites.

Spoon the mixture lightly into the prepared loaf tin and bake for 35–40 minutes, or until golden brown.

Let the loaf cool in the tin.

When the loaf is completely cold, remove it from the tin and wrap it in foil. Let it stand for 24 hours, then unwrap it and cut it into wafer-thin slices (use a sharp, serrated-edge knife).

INGREDIENTS

155 g (5 oz)
plain (all-purpose) flour

¼ teaspoon cinnamon

3 egg whites

½ cup (125 g, 4 oz) sugar

60 g (2 oz)
whole raw almonds

60 g (2 oz) whole Brazil nuts,
lightly chopped

Place the slices on a sheet of non-stick baking parchment on a baking tray (sheet) and bake at 120°C (250°F) for 30–35 minutes, or until dry and crisp.

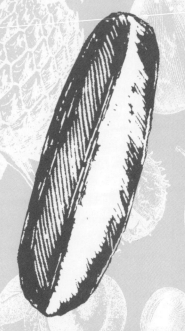

Let the slices cool completely, then store them in an airtight container and serve with coffee or tea or as an accompaniment to desserts.

Serves 12 to 18

Mediterranean Clove Cookies

S
W
E
E
T

H
E
A
L
T
H

Line 2 baking sheets (trays) with non-stick baking parchment. Lightly dust the baking parchment with cornflour.

Sift the icing sugar with the cloves.

Place the egg whites and icing sugar in a mixing bowl and whip (use an electric beater) until the mixture is stiff and fluffy. Fold the sifted flour through the egg whites, stopping as soon as the flour is incorporated.

Let the mixture rest, covered with a damp cloth, for 1 hour.

Knead the rested dough on a lightly floured bench surface. Keep the dough and your hands lightly floured to prevent stickiness.

Form heaped spoonfuls of the mixture into pear shapes using well floured hands. Use up all the mixture. Then make three cuts down one side of each cookie, using a pair of scissors. Place the cookies on the prepared trays, bending them slightly to open up the cuts.

INGREDIENTS

a little cornflour (cornstarch)

1⅓ cups (250 g, 8 oz) icing (powdered) sugar

¼ teaspoon ground cloves

5 egg whites

2¼ cups (280 g, 9 oz) plain (all-purpose) flour, sifted

icing (powdered) sugar, extra, for dusting

Let the cookies sit, uncovered, at room temperature for 8–10 hours (or overnight).

Preheat the oven to 200°C (400°F).

Bake the cookies for 10–12 minutes, or until they are a light golden brown.

Remove from the oven and cool before dusting lightly with icing sugar and storing in an airtight container. The cookies will keep this way for 1–2 weeks.

Makes 24 to 30

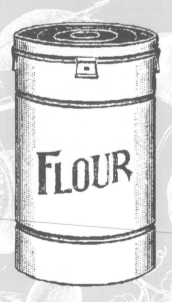

Sauterne and Citrus Jellies

Place the sauterne, orange juice, cinnamon sticks, sugar and gelatine in a saucepan. Leave for several minutes so that the gelatine can soak.

Bring the liquid to the boil over a medium heat, stirring frequently. As soon as the mixture boils, remove the saucepan from the heat. Remove the cinnamon sticks and let the liquid cool to room temperature. Place the cooled liquid in the refrigerator to thicken (do not let it set).

Place 1–2 tablespoons of the liquid into each of 6 dariole moulds. Place these in the refrigerator to set firm (20–30 minutes). When the jelly is firm, layer slices of orange and grapefruit onto it, then cover with the remaining jelly.

Return the jellies to the refrigerator and chill until they are set firm (about 1 hour). To unmould, dip the base of each mould into a bowl of hot water for 1–2 seconds. Turn the jellies out onto serving plates covered with fresh fruit or a berry sauce.

Serves 6

INGREDIENTS

SAUTERNE AND CITRUS JELLIES

2 cups (500 mL, 16 fl oz) sauterne

1 cup (250 mL, 8 fl oz) orange juice

2 cinnamon sticks

¼ cup (60 g, 2 oz) sugar

30 g (1 oz) powdered gelatine

1 cup (250 g, 8 oz) orange segments

1 cup (250 g, 8 oz) grapefruit segments

fresh fruit or berry sauce, for serving

ZABAGLIONE

6 egg yolks

¼ cup (60 mL, 2 fl oz) Grand Marnier

½ cup (125 g, 4 oz) sugar

zest of 1 orange, finely grated

1 cup (250 mL, 8 fl oz) double (heavy, thickened) cream, whipped

Zabaglione

Beat the sugar and egg yolks with the orange zest and Grand Marnier in a large stainless steel bowl until the mixture begins to lighten in colour and becomes aerated. Place the bowl over a bain-marie (water bath) and whisk constantly until the mixture is frothy and thick, and has doubled in volume. The mixture should be able to hold its shape when drizzled over itself.

Allow the whisked egg mixture to cook slightly, but be very careful not to curdle or overcook it. Fold through the whipped cream.

Pour the zabaglione into tall champagne or parfait glasses, then chill and serve.

Serves 4

Honey Slice

INGREDIENTS

½ cup (185 g, 6 oz)
clear honey

2 tablespoons golden syrup
(light treacle)

6 tablespoons walnut oil

½ cup (125 g, 4 oz) sugar

3 cups (375 g, 12 oz)
plain (all-purpose) flour

1 teaspoon ground cinnamon

2 teaspoons baking powder
(soda)

1⅓ cups (155 g, 5 oz)
ground almonds

2 eggs

juice and finely grated zest
of 1 lemon

HONEY GLAZE

2 tablespoons clear honey

1 tablespoon lemon juice

1 cup (185 g, 6 oz)
icing (powdered) sugar

Grease a 28 x 18 x 2 cm (11 x 7 x ¾ in) baking tray (jelly roll pan) and line the base with non-stick baking parchment.

Place the honey, golden syrup, oil and sugar in a saucepan and bring to the boil. Stir the mixture occasionally to make sure it doesn't burn. Boil for 2 minutes.

Remove the saucepan from the heat and let the mixture cool.

Sift the flour, cinnamon and baking powder into a bowl, then add the ground almonds and eggs.

Add the cooled liquid and work the mixture with a spoon until it forms a dough.

Remove the dough from the bowl and press it by hand into the tray. Refrigerate the dough for 2 hours.

Preheat the oven to 180°C (350°F).

Bake the slice for 45 minutes, or until a skewer inserted into the top comes out clean.

Remove from the oven and glaze immediately. You may not need to use all the glaze.

Cool the slice before cutting. If the glaze doesn't set after 1 hour, place the slice in the refrigerator for 40–50 minutes.

Cut into very thin slices and serve for afternoon teas, snacks, or with coffee.

TO MAKE THE HONEY GLAZE

Place the honey and lemon juice in a bowl. Slowly mix in the icing sugar until it is all combined and no lumps remain. Leftover glaze should be thrown away, as it will not keep.

Serves 10 to 12

Bitter Marmalade Cake

Preheat the oven to 180°C (350°F). Lightly grease a 23 cm (9 in) springform cake tin and cover its base with a disc of non-stick baking parchment.

Place the oranges in a large saucepan, cover them with water and bring to the boil. Boil the oranges for 1½ hours, then place them in a blender or food processor (while they are still hot) and blend to a pulp.

Beat the egg yolks with half of the sugar, until the mixture is thick and fluffy.

Beat the egg whites until they form stiff peaks. Gradually add the remaining sugar, a spoonful at a time, beating well after each addition, until all the sugar is dissolved.

Stir the baking powder and ground almonds into the egg yolk mixture, then add the orange pulp. Gently fold through the egg whites.

INGREDIENTS

3 whole oranges

6 egg yolks

¾ cup (185 g, 6 oz) caster (superfine) sugar

8 egg whites

1 teaspoon baking powder (soda)

2½ cups (280 g, 9 oz) ground almonds

icing (powdered) sugar, for dusting

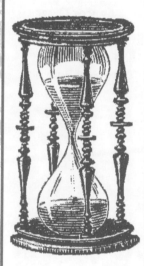

Pour the mixture into the prepared tin and bake for 55–60 minutes, or until the cake has shrunk from the sides of the tin slightly and the top springs back after being touched.

Let the cake cool in the tin. When the cake is cold, remove it from the tin, dust it lightly with icing sugar, then serve.

Serves 8 to 10

Flourless Walnut Cake

Preheat the oven to 180°C (350°F). Lightly grease a 23 cm (9 in) springform cake tin and line it with non-stick baking parchment.

In a large bowl, whisk the egg yolks, cinnamon and sugar until they are thick, and light in colour.

In a separate bowl, whisk the egg whites until they form stiff peaks. Gradually add the sugar, a spoonful at a time, beating well after each addition. Continue whisking until the sugar is incorporated and dissolved.

Add the melted chocolate to the egg yolk mixture and combine well.

Working quickly, so that the chocolate does not tighten as it cools, fold half of the egg white mixture into the chocolate mixture and combine thoroughly.

Fold through the walnuts, orange zest and the remaining egg whites, then pour the mixture into the prepared cake tin. Bake until the cake is firm in the centre, about 45–50 minutes. Remove the cake from the oven and let it cool in the tin. Then run a sharp knife around the inside edge of the tin and remove the cake.

To Make the Apricot Glaze

Place the apricot jam, water and lemon juice in a small saucepan and bring to the boil, stirring constantly.

Boil the mixture for 4–5 minutes, until the bubbles become very small and the mixture is syrupy.

Remove the syrup from the heat and let it cool slightly, then glaze the cake thoroughly. Let the cake cool before serving in thin slices with tea or coffee.

Serves 8 to 10

INGREDIENTS

5 egg yolks

¼ teaspoon cinnamon

90 g (3 oz) sugar

5 egg whites

90 g (3 oz) sugar

225 g (7 oz) dark (plain or semi-sweet) chocolate, melted

225 g (7 oz) ground walnuts

finely grated zest of 1 orange

APRICOT GLAZE

185 g (6 oz) apricot jam

¼ cup (60 mL, 2 fl oz) water

2 teaspoons lemon juice

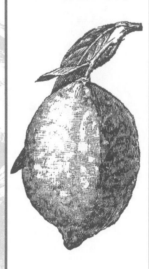

Beetroot Cake

Preheat the oven to 180°C (350°F). Lightly grease a 23 cm (9 in) springform cake tin and line its base with non-stick baking parchment.

Sift the flour, baking powder and cinnamon.

In a large bowl, whisk the egg yolks with the sugar until light, thick and fluffy.

Gently fold through the beetroot, almonds, hazelnuts, breadcrumbs and sifted dry ingredients.

In a separate bowl, whisk the egg whites until they form stiff peaks. Fold the egg whites through the egg yolk mixture. Pour the mixture into the tin and bake until the cake has shrunk away from the sides of the pan, about 30–35 minutes.

Cool in the tin on a wire rack.

When the cake is completely cold, turn it out onto a serving platter and dust lightly with icing sugar.

Serves 8 to 10

BEETROOT CAKE

½ cup (60 g, 2 oz) plain (all-purpose) flour

1 teaspoon baking powder (soda)

1 teaspoon cinnamon

7 egg yolks

¾ cup (185 g, 6 oz) sugar

185 g (6 oz) fresh beetroot, finely grated

90 g (3 oz) ground almonds

75 g (2½ oz) ground hazelnuts

45 g (1½ oz) dry breadcrumbs

7 egg whites

icing (powdered) sugar, for dusting

CHOCOLATE CHIP MUFFINS

3¼ cups (405 g, 13 oz) plain (all-purpose) flour

1 tablespoon baking powder (soda)

¾ cup (125 g, 4 oz) brown sugar (light)

½ cup (125 g, 4 oz) sugar

125 g (4 oz) chocolate chips

2½ cups (125 g, 4 oz) shredded coconut

1¼ cups (310 mL, 10 fl oz) soy milk

⅓ cup (75 mL, 2½ oz) olive oil

2 eggs, lightly beaten

Chocolate Chip Muffins

Preheat the oven to 180°C (350°F). Lightly grease a 12-cup muffin tray.

Sift the flour and baking powder into a large bowl. Add the sugars, chocolate chips and coconut. Stir lightly to combine.

Add the soy milk, oil and eggs. Mix until all ingredients are moist.

Three-quarters fill all the cups on the muffin tray and bake for 25–30 minutes, or until the muffins are firm in the centre when touched.

Let the muffins cool for 5 minutes in the tray, then place them on a cooling rack. Serve warm or cold.

Makes 12

Chocolate Sauce

Place the water, sugar and chocolate in a saucepan and slowly bring to the boil, stirring continuously.

Mix the extra water with the cocoa, cornflour and extra sugar. Whisk lightly to remove any lumps.

When the first mixture has boiled, slowly add the second mixture. Let the sauce come to the boil again, stirring continuously.

Remove from the heat. The sauce can be served hot, immediately, or allowed to cool and served cold.

**Makes 2½ cups
(625 mL, 20 fl oz)**

INGREDIENTS

CHOCOLATE SAUCE

1 cup (250 mL, 8 fl oz) water

½ cup (125 g, 4 oz) sugar

60 g (2 oz) dark
(plain or semi-sweet)
chocolate, chopped

½ cup (125 mL, 4 fl oz)
water, extra

45 g (1½ oz) unsweetened
cocoa powder, sifted

1 tablespoon cornflour
(cornstarch), sifted

⅓ cup (90 g, 3 oz) sugar,
extra

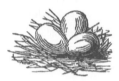

GELATO

1½ cups (375 g, 12 oz) sugar

1 cup (250 mL, 8 fl oz)
fresh orange juice

4 cups (1 litre, 32 fl oz)
water

3 egg whites

½ cup (90 g, 3 oz)
icing (powdered) sugar

Gelato

Place the sugar, orange juice and water in a large saucepan and bring slowly to the boil.

Boil for 15 minutes, uncovered.

Let the mixture cool, then pour it into a large baking tray (jelly roll pan). Freeze the mixture for 24 hours.

In a large bowl of an electric mixer, whisk the egg whites and icing sugar to a firm meringue (stiff peaks).

Remove the frozen ice, break it up finely (use a whisk), add it to the meringue and whisk thoroughly until combined.

Freeze the mixture for a further 6 hours before serving.

Serves 6 to 8

Blueberry Pie

Put the flour and sugar into a bowl and rub the margarine through until the mixture has the consistency of breadcrumbs.

Add the egg yolk and water and mix to a dough. Remove the dough and knead it lightly, then wrap it in plastic wrap (cling film) and refrigerate it for 20 minutes.

Lightly oil a 20 cm (8 in) deep pie dish.

Cut off two-thirds of the pastry to use, and refrigerate the remaining third.

On a lightly floured bench surface, roll the dough so that it fits into the base of the pie dish. Line the pie dish with the pastry. Refrigerate until the base is required.

2¾ cups (225 g, 7 oz) plain (all-purpose) flour

1 teaspoon caster (superfine) sugar

100 g (3½ oz) milk-free margarine

1 egg yolk

½ cup (125 mL, 4 fl oz) water

FILLING

500 g (1 lb) blueberries

3 tablespoons orange juice

finely grated zest of 1 orange

¼ teaspoon cinnamon

2 tablespoons cornflour (cornstarch)

2 tablespoons brown sugar (light)

1 egg white, lightly whisked

2 tablespoons sugar, extra

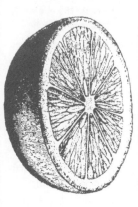

To Make the Filling

Preheat the oven to 200°C (400°F).

Wash the berries, then, in a large bowl, mix them with the orange juice and zest, cinnamon, cornflour and sugar.

Place the berry mixture on top of the pie base.

Roll the remaining chilled pastry on a lightly floured bench surface and drape it over the top of the pie.

Brush the top of the pie lightly with the egg white, then sprinkle lightly with the extra sugar.

Bake the pie until the top and the base (check by inserting a knife between the crust and the pie dish) look golden brown, about 40 minutes.

Let the pie cool slightly before serving, or serve it cold.

Serves 6 to 8

Wholemeal Spice and Lemon Cake

Preheat the oven to 180°C (350°F). Lightly grease an 18 x 7 x 5 cm (7 x 3 x 2 in) loaf tin and line it with non-stick baking parchment.

Sift the flour into a mixing bowl, reserving the bran for later use. Stir in the cinnamon, mixed spice, baking powder and bicarbonate of soda.

In a small saucepan, heat the golden syrup and the margarine until they become liquid.

Add the golden syrup mixture, soya milk and lemon zest to the flour mixture and stir well.

Pour the cake batter into the loaf tin. Sprinkle the remainder of the bran on top of the mixture.

Bake for 70–80 minutes, or until a toothpick inserted into the cake comes out clean.

Let the cake cool in the tin. Serve the cake in thin slices with coffee.

Serves 8 to 10

INGREDIENTS

WHOLEMEAL SPICE AND LEMON CAKE

1¾ cups (225 g, 7 oz) wholemeal (whole-wheat) plain flour

½ teaspoon cinnamon

½ teaspoon mixed spice

1 teaspoon baking powder (soda)

⅓ teaspoon bicarbonate of soda

½ cup (185 g, 6 oz) golden syrup (light treacle)

100 g (3½ oz) milk-free margarine

¼ cup (60 mL, 2 fl oz) soy milk

finely grated zest of 1 lemon

BOILED FRUIT CAKE

1 cup (185 g, 6 oz) brown sugar (light)

1½ cups (185 g, 6 oz) chopped walnuts

¾ cup (90 g, 3 oz) chopped blanched almonds

30 g (1 oz) milk-free margarine

1 teaspoon cinnamon

¼ teaspoon nutmeg

1 cup (250 mL, 8 fl oz) water

1 cup (185 g, 6 oz) sultanas (golden raisins)

1½ cups (250 g, 8 oz) glacé cherries

1 teaspoon bicarbonate of soda

2 tablespoons water, extra

2 cups (250 g, 8 oz) plain (all-purpose) flour

1 tablespoon baking powder (soda)

Boiled Fruit Cake

Preheat the oven to 180°C (350°F). Lightly oil a 20 cm (8 in) springform cake tin and line its base with non-stick baking parchment.

Place the sugar, nuts, margarine, spices, water and fruit in a large saucepan and slowly bring to the boil, stirring constantly.

Boil for 4 minutes, then remove from the heat and leave to cool.

Dissolve the bicarbonate of soda in the water and add it to the fruit mixture.

In a bowl, sift the flour with the baking powder, then fold in the fruit mixture.

Place the mixture in the tin and bake for 60–90 minutes.

Let the cake cool in the tin. When it is cold, wrap it in foil and store till required. The cake will keep this way for 1–2 weeks.

Serves 8 to 10

Sweet or Savoury Bread Rolls

Line two baking trays (sheets) with non-stick baking parchment.

Sift the flour into a bowl, then add the sugar and salt.

Dissolve the yeast in the soy milk.

Mix the margarine into the flour until the mixture has the consistency of fine breadcrumbs.

Add the milk and yeast to the flour mix and work to a dough.

Remove the dough from the bowl and knead heavily against the bench surface for 5–8 minutes. By this time the dough should be smooth, and not sticky.

Return the dough to a lightly floured bowl, cover with a damp cloth and leave to rise in a warm place for about 45 minutes, or until it has doubled in size.

INGREDIENTS

3½ cups (435 g, 14 oz) plain (all-purpose) flour

1 tablespoon sugar

½ teaspoon salt

15 g (½ oz) fresh compressed yeast

1⅓ cups (310 mL, 10 fl oz) soy milk

60 g (2 oz) milk-free margarine

Turn the dough out of the bowl and divide it into 24 equal portions. Knead the portions into small balls and leave to prove (rise) for 30 minutes, or until it has doubled in size.

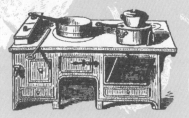

Preheat the oven to 200°C (400°F).

Bake the buns for 15–20 minutes, then leave them to cool.

Serve the buns with jam or savoury fillings for dessert, snacks or lunch.

Makes 24

Steamed Fruit Pudding

Lightly oil (or grease with milk-free margarine) a 1½ –2 litre (2½–3¼ imp. pint) pudding basin.

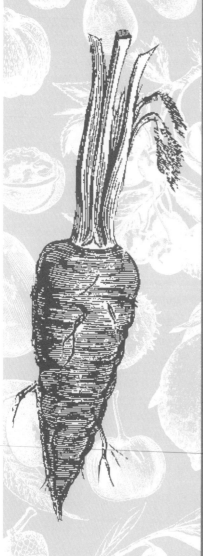

INGREDIENTS

¾ cup (90 g, 3 oz) plain (all-purpose) flour

½ teaspoon cinnamon

¼ teaspoon ground cloves

1¼ cups (225 g, 7 oz) brown sugar (light)

½ cup (60 g, 2 oz) dry breadcrumbs

100 g (3½ oz) shredded suet

1 cup (185 g, 6 oz) raisins

1 cup (155 g, 5 oz) currants

185 g (6 oz) grated carrot

185 g (6 oz) grated raw potato

juice and finely grated zest of 1 lemon

2 eggs, lightly beaten

1 cup (155 g, 5 oz) mixed (candied) peel

1 teaspoon bicarbonate of soda

½ cup (125 mL, 4 fl oz) warm water

light citrus sauce, for serving (see page 64)

Sift the flour, cinnamon and cloves into a large bowl.

Stir in the sugar, breadcrumbs and suet.

In a separate bowl, mix together the currants, raisins, grated carrot and potato, lemon juice and zest, eggs and mixed peel.

In a small bowl, mix the bicarbonate of soda with the water. Add this to the carrot mixture and mix together until thoroughly combined. Add this mixture to the sifted dry ingredients.

Pour the mixture into the pudding basin, cover tightly with non-stick baking parchment and a lid (or foil) and steam the pudding for 2½–3 hours.

Serve small portions of this heavy fruited pudding with a light citrus sauce.

Serves 6 to 8

Lemon Snow

Place the caster sugar and water in a saucepan and bring to the boil.

Mix the cornflour with the lemon juice to make a smooth paste.

When the water boils, remove the saucepan from the heat and whisk in the lemon/cornflour mixture. Return to the heat and stir constantly until the mixture reboils.

Remove from the heat and leave to cool.

In a separate bowl, whisk the egg whites until they form stiff peaks. Gently fold the egg whites through the cooling lemon mixture. Refrigerate the mixture until it is cold (and has thickened) and serve, on its own.

Serves 4 to 6

LEMON SNOW

1 cup (225 g, 7 oz) caster (superfine) sugar

2 cups (500 mL, 16 fl oz) water

2 tablespoons cornflour (cornstarch)

juice and finely grated zest of 2 lemons

2 egg whites

PEAR CAKE

2 eggs

1 cup (250 mL, 8 fl oz) olive oil

1½ cups (375 g, 12 oz) sugar

1 teaspoon vanilla

1 teaspoon bicarbonate of soda

2 teaspoons water

2 cups (250 g, 8 oz) plain (all-purpose) flour

2 teaspoons cinnamon

3 large pears, peeled and cut into 1 cm (½ in) dice

icing (powdered) sugar, for dusting

Pear Cake

Preheat the oven to 180°C (350°F). Line the base of a 20 cm (8 in) springform cake tin with non-stick baking parchment.

In a large bowl, whisk the eggs and oil until foamy.

Add the sugar, vanilla, bicarbonate of soda and water and beat until light and fluffy.

Add the flour and cinnamon and beat until smooth.

Fold through the pear pieces.

Spread the mixture in the base of the prepared tin.

Bake for 60–65 minutes, or until a toothpick inserted into the middle of the cake comes out clean.

Cool the cake in the tin. When it is cold, dust it with icing sugar and serve.

Serves 8 to 10

107

L A C T O S E F R E E D E S S E R T S

Salt-free and Low-salt Desserts

In today's world of manufactured and preprocessed foods the intake of salt per person has increased, becoming a major health problem. Too much salt in our diet increases the risk of hypertension (high blood pressure), which can lead to heart disease, stroke and kidney failure.

While the increase of salt in the diet is sometimes caused by the heavyhandedness of the home cook or chef, salt also comes already supplied in many of the manufactured goods that we use in our cooking. Every opportunity should be taken to reduce the amount of salt in the diet, especially in the foods we prepare at home.

Foods high in salt include preserved meat, takeaway foods, snack foods such as potato chips, preserved vegetables, spreads (e.g. Vegemite), packet soups, stock cubes, baking soda, canned or processed foods and meat tenderisers.

The home cook and chef who is working to a low-salt or no-salt diet must check food labels, in the same way that those who are on a low-cholesterol or low-fat diet or have an intolerance to sugar or gluten do. Other names for common salt to look for are sodium chloride, vegetable/sea salt and monosodium glutamate.

To understand the need to reduce the amount of salt we eat, we must understand the role salt plays in the body. The body requires a fine balance of fluid both inside and outside its cells. Sodium is responsible for part of this, maintaining fluid levels both between and outside the cells. Potassium maintains the level of fluids inside the cells.

In a healthy body the ratio of potassium to salt is in perfect harmony, and the body's fluid levels are maintained and regulated by the kidneys. When we have an excess of sodium, however, it has to be excreted by our kidneys. To do this, water is retained to dilute the sodium to the normal concentration. The blood volume in the arteries therefore increases and blood pressure is raised slightly until the excess sodium and fluid are excreted. Continuing to eat a diet high in salt could permanently increase your blood pressure. Because the kidneys are the regulators of the sodium balance, kidney failure is also a major risk.

However, while high salt intake is a contributing factor to heart attack and strokes, it is not the sole cause. A diet high in sodium is often also high in saturated fats and inadequate in fibre.

The best way to reduce salt is to eat foods which have either no salt content or a very low salt content.

For most people, cooking without using salt would be a good thing. Other ways to reduce the amount of salt you eat are to eat more freshly-prepared foods, making more use of herbs and spices, and checking the labels of foods you buy for added salt.

If you have high sodium levels in your body, or any of the symptoms of high salt levels, you are probably already on a restricted-salt diet. These recipes can just be substituted into your food plan.

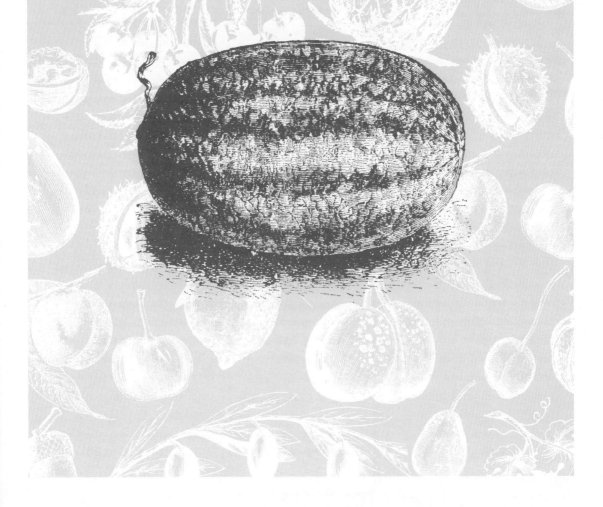

Chocolate Mocha Custard

Preheat the oven to 180°C (350°F).

Place the milk, sugar and coffee granules in a saucepan and bring slowly to the boil. Add the chocolate and stir through thoroughly.

In a bowl, beat the eggs with the first amount of butter. Pour the boiled liquid over this and whisk well to combine.

In a frypan (skillet), melt the extra butter over a low heat, then add the extra sugar. Stir the mixture constantly for 3–5 minutes, until the sugar melts and the mixture turns golden brown, then stir in the breadcrumbs and cinnamon.

Cook the mixture for 1–2 minutes, then remove it from the heat and let it cool.

Line a deep quiche (pie) dish with the breadcrumb mixture, then pour the custard over it. Do not worry if the breadcrumbs float or mix with the custard. Bake in a water bath for about 1 hour, or until set. Let the custard cool for 20 minutes, then serve with sponge fingers and cream.

Serves 4 to 6

INGREDIENTS

CHOCOLATE MOCHA CUSTARD

2 cups (500 mL, 16 fl oz) milk

3 tablespoons sugar

2 tablespoons instant coffee granules

60 g (2 oz) dark (plain or semi-sweet) chocolate, melted

2 eggs

6 teaspoons unsalted butter, melted

1 tablespoon unsalted butter, extra

2 tablespoons sugar, extra

⅔ cup (75 g, 2½ oz) dry breadcrumbs

1 teaspoon ground cinnamon

sponge fingers (see below) and cream, for serving

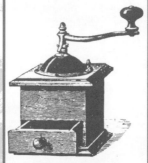

SPONGE FINGERS

⅔ cup (90 g, 3 oz) cornflour (cornstarch)

⅓ cup (90 g, 3 oz) sugar

5 egg yolks

75 g (2½ oz) sugar, extra

½ teaspoon ground cinnamon

3 egg whites

⅔ cup (75 g, 2½ oz) plain (all-purpose) flour

Sponge Fingers

Preheat the oven to 180°C (350°F). Line 3 baking trays (sheets) with non-stick baking parchment.

Combine the cornflour and sugar. Use half of the mixture to lightly dust the lined baking tray. Reserve the remaining mixture.

In a bowl, whisk the egg yolks, extra sugar and cinnamon until thick, light and fluffy. In another bowl, whisk the egg whites until they form stiff peaks.

Fold the flour through the egg yolk mixture and then lightly fold in the egg whites.

Using a 0.5 cm (⅛ in) plain piping nozzle attached to a piping (pastry) bag, pipe 10 cm (4 in) fingers onto the prepared tray.

Dust the tops of the fingers very lightly with the remaining cornflour and sugar mixture, then bake for 12–15 minutes, or until golden brown.

Let the sponge fingers cool on the tray. When they are cold, store them in an airtight container.

Makes 18 to 24

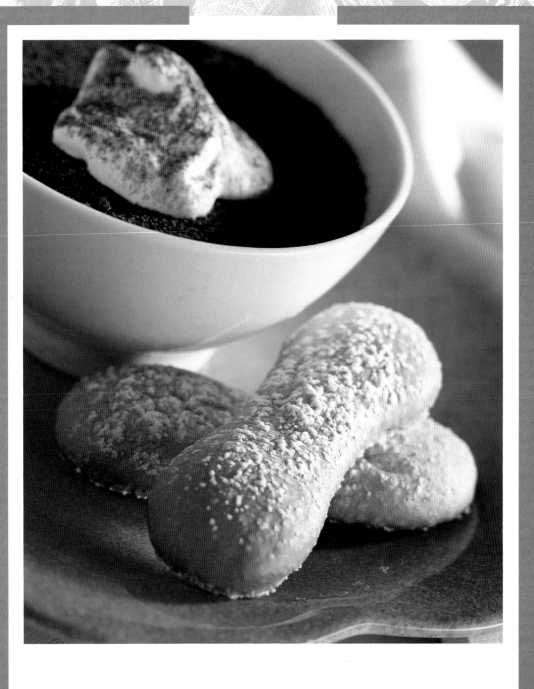

Chocolate Mocha Custard and Sponge Fingers

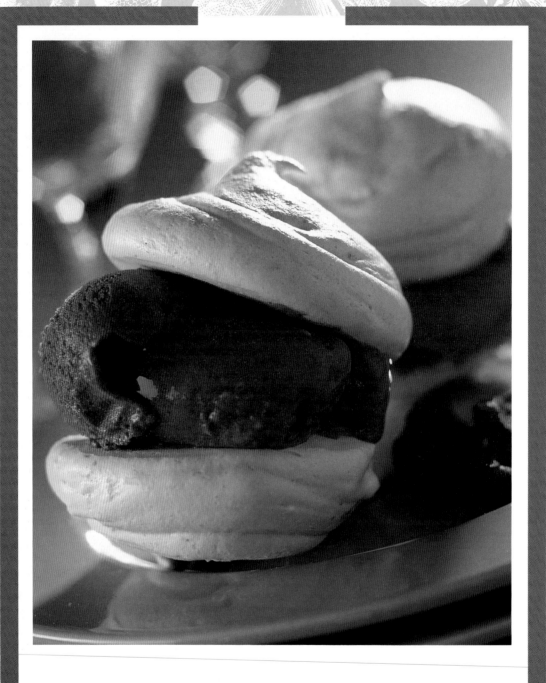

Meringue Kisses and Raspberry Sorbet (page 114)

Meringue Kisses

Preheat the oven to 120°C (250°F). Line a baking sheet (tray) with non-stick baking parchment and dust this lightly with cornflour (cornstarch).

Whisk the egg whites until they form stiff peaks. Gradually add the sugar, a tablespoon at a time, beating well after each addition. Whisk until the sugar is completely dissolved and incorporated.

Fold through the icing sugar and the macadamia nuts.

Spoon tablespoons of the meringue mixture onto the baking tray. Dust them lightly with icing sugar and bake them for 45–50 minutes. Turn the oven off and let the meringues finish cooking in the dying heat.

Serve the meringues cold as a dessert or as an afternoon tea treat with marinated fruits, chocolate mousse or whipped cream.

Serves 4 to 6

INGREDIENTS

MERINGUE KISSES

a little cornflour (cornstarch)

3 egg whites

⅔ cup (155 g, 5 oz) sugar

1 teaspoon icing (powdered) sugar, sifted

30 g (1 oz) macadamia (Queensland) nuts, chopped and roasted

marinated fruit, or chocolate mousse, or whipped cream, for serving

SOUR CREAM AND PEANUT MUFFINS

6 eggs

4 tablespoons sour cream

4 tablespoons unsalted butter, melted

1 cup (125 g, 4 oz) plain (all-purpose) flour, sifted

2 teaspoons sodium-free baking powder (soda) (see page 121)

1 tablespoon sugar

1 teaspoon bicarbonate of soda

4 tablespoons peanut butter (salt-free)

1 teaspoon cinnamon

Sour Cream and Peanut Muffins

Preheat the oven to 180°C (350°F). Grease a 12 cup muffin tray.

Place the eggs, sour cream and butter in a bowl and whisk thoroughly. Add the flour, baking powder, sugar, peanut butter and bicarbonate of soda. Beat the mixture well, until smooth.

Pour the mixture into the 12 muffin cups and bake for 35–45 minutes. Let the muffins cool in the tray for 5–10 minutes, then remove them. Serve warm or cold.

Makes 12 muffins

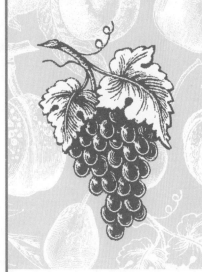

Raspberry Sorbet

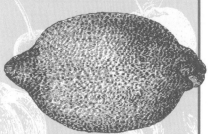

INGREDIENTS

1 kg (2 lb) raspberries
2 tablespoons Grand Marnier
2 tablespoons liquid glucose
(corn syrup)
juice of 1 lemon
1 egg white

Place the raspberries in a blender or food processor and purée until they form a fine pulp.

Sieve the purée to remove the seeds and separate the juice.

Place the purée in a saucepan with the Grand Marnier, glucose and lemon juice and bring slowly to the boil.

When the mixture is boiling, remove it from the heat and let it cool.

Place the cooled mixture in a container and freeze to the point where it is mushy and small ice particles have formed (1–2 hours). Stir it occasionally with a fork during the freezing process.

Whisk the egg white until it forms stiff peaks.

Fold the egg white into the lightly frozen raspberry mixture.

Refreeze the sorbet and stir it briskly for 2–3 minutes every hour. Let the mixture freeze for 4 hours before leaving to freeze overnight. Serve as an accompaniment to a light or rich dessert or on its own as a light, healthy snack.

Serves 4 to 6

Shortbread

INGREDIENTS

4 cups (500 g, 16 oz)
plain (all-purpose) flour
310 g (10 oz) unsalted butter
⅔ cup (155 g, 5 oz) sugar
sugar, extra, for dusting

Preheat the oven to 180°C (350°F). Line 2 baking trays (sheets) with non-stick baking parchment.

Place all the ingredients in a mixing bowl. Using your fingertips, crumb the butter through the dry ingredients, until the mixture has the consistency of fresh breadcrumbs.

Scrape the mixture down and continue working until a dough is formed.

Knead the dough lightly, then press it evenly onto the tray, right to the edges.

Use a fork to form a pattern of holes on the top of the shortbread.

Use a knife to mark (quite deeply) the lines along which the shortbread is to be cut after cooking.

Bake the shortbread for 25 minutes, or until it is golden brown around the edges and lightly brown on top.

Remove from the oven and sprinkle with some of the extra sugar.

Let the shortbread cool, then cut it and remove it from the tray. Sprinkle each piece with sugar again and store in an airtight container. They will keep for 1–2 weeks.

Serves 18 to 24

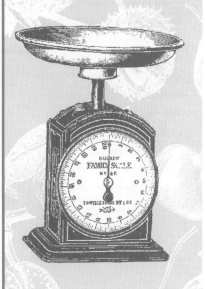

Cherry Soup

In a saucepan, combine the cherries, water, cinnamon stick, lemon and cloves.

Bring this mixture to the boil, then simmer for 15 minutes. Strain the liquid into a large measuring jug. Remove the cinnamon stick and the cloves, then press the pulp through a sieve into the jug as well.

Add enough water to make the mixture up to 4 cups, then pour the soup back into the saucepan. Stir in the sugar, lemon and orange juice and tapioca.

Bring to the boil, then simmer for about 10 minutes, or until the tapioca is transparent.

Chill the soup for at least 4 hours.

INGREDIENTS

4 cups pitted sweet black cherries

1 cup (250 mL, 8 fl oz) water

1 cinnamon stick

1 lemon, thinly sliced

6 whole cloves

¼ cup (60 g, 2 oz) sugar

juice of 1 lemon

juice of 1 orange

2 teaspoons tapioca

nutmeg or grated chocolate, for decoration

Serve in icy cold bowls, with a dollop of sour cream and a sprinkling of nutmeg or chocolate, as a first course or as dessert.

Serves 4

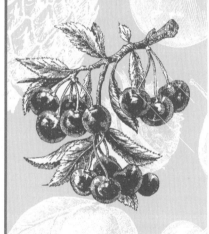

Apricot and Apple Torte

To Make the Base

Put the wheatgerm, coconut and sesame seeds into a blender or food processor and grind for 2 minutes. During this 2 minutes, add the melted butter. Process until combined.

Line a 20 cm (8 in) springform cake tin with non-stick baking parchment. Press the mixture evenly over the base of the tin. Place the base in the refrigerator until required.

To Make the Filling

Peel and core the apples, then cut them into thin slices. Place the apple and the dried apricots in a saucepan with the orange zest and juice and cook over a low heat until the liquid has been absorbed. Remove from the heat and leave to cool.

Base

1 cup (125 g, 4 oz) wheatgerm

⅓ cup (30 g, 1 oz) freshly grated coconut

¼ cup (60 g, 2 oz) sesame seeds

60 g (2 oz) unsalted butter, melted

Filling

6 medium green cooking (Granny Smith) apples

½ cup (60 g, 2 oz) finely chopped dried apricots

zest of 1 orange, finely grated

1 cup (250 mL, 8 fl oz) orange juice

Topping

30 g (1 oz) flaked almonds

60 g (2 oz) rolled oats (minute, quick cooking)

1 teaspoon cinnamon

2 tablespoons raw sugar

60 g (2 oz) unsalted butter

To Make the Topping

Place all the topping ingredients except the butter on a baking tray (sheet) and toast lightly in the oven until the nuts are golden brown (5–8 minutes).

To Assemble the Cake

Spoon the warm apple mixture over the chilled base and smooth down. Sprinkle the toasted mixture evenly over the top of the apple and press down with the base of a spoon. Cut the unsalted butter into small pieces and sprinkle them on top of the topping mixture.

Bake for about 45 minutes.

Remove the torte from the oven, let it cool on a wire rack, then refrigerate it overnight. Before serving, remove the torte from the tin.

Serves 10

Pancake Fruit Stack

INGREDIENTS

2 cups (250 g, 8 oz)
plain (all-purpose) flour

4 teaspoons sodium-free
baking powder (soda)
(see page 121)

1 teaspoon cinnamon

½ cup (60 g, 2 oz) buckwheat

2 egg whites

½–¾ cup (125–185 mL,
4–6 fl oz) milk

FILLING

500 g (1 lb) fresh apricot,
peach or pear halves

1 cup (250 mL, 8 fl oz)
fresh orange juice

zest of 1 orange

250 g (8 oz) cottage cheese

TO MAKE THE PANCAKES

In a bowl, whisk together all
the pancake ingredients. Use
only ½ cup (125 mL, 4 fl oz) of
milk at first, then keep adding
until desired consistency
(thick but pourable) is
obtained.

Pour 3–4 tablespoons of the
mixture into a non-stick
frypan (skillet) and cook until
bubbles appear on the
upturned side. Turn over (use
a spatula) and cook the other
side until golden brown. Place
the cooked pancakes on a
plate or a tray lined with foil
and cover them to keep them
warm. Keep cooking until all
mixture has been used.

TO MAKE THE FILLING

Place the fruit, orange juice
and zest in a saucepan and
heat gently until the mixture
comes to a simmer. Simmer
for 5 minutes, until the volume
of the liquid has been
considerably reduced and the
fruit is tender.

TO ASSEMBLE THE PANCAKE STACK

Spread each pancake with
cottage cheese, then make the
stack. Start with a pancake,
then pour over some of the
fruit mixture, then add another
pancake, then more fruit
mixture and so on, until all
pancakes have been used.

Pour any remaining fruit
mixture over the top of the
pancake stack and bring the
stack, warm, to the table. Give
each person a knife to cut a
slice from the pancake stack.

Serves 8 to 10

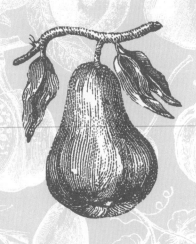

Scotch Black Bun

Preheat the oven to 180°C (350°F).

Mix the bran, currants and milk in a bowl. Cover and leave to stand in the refrigerator overnight.

Sift the flour and baking powder together, then add the chopped walnuts, cinnamon and cloves.

Add the flour mixture to the fruit and bran mixture and beat well.

Lightly grease a 20 x 8 x 7 cm (8 x 3 x 3 in) loaf tin. Line its base with non-stick baking parchment. Spread the mixture evenly into the tin and bake for 55–60 minutes.

Leave the bun to cool for 30–40 minutes, then serve in thin slices.

Serves 8 to 10

SCOTCH BLACK BUN

1 cup (125 g, 4 oz) bran

1 cup (155 g, 5 oz) currants (salt-free)

2 cups (500 mL, 16 fl oz) milk

1½ cups (185 g, 6 oz) plain (all-purpose) flour

2 teaspoons sodium-free baking powder (soda) (see page 121)

¼ cup (30 g, 1 oz) chopped walnuts

½ teaspoon ground cinnamon

¼ teaspoon ground cloves

ENGLISH AFTERNOON TEA LEMON CAKE

½ cup (125 mL, 4 fl oz) single (light, whipping) cream

1 cup (125 g, 4 oz) plain (all-purpose) flour

1½ teaspoons sodium-free baking powder (soda) (see page 121)

3 eggs

6 teaspoons sugar

juice and zest of 1 lemon

citrus sauce (see page 64) or cream, for serving

English Afternoon Tea Lemon Cake

Preheat the oven to 160°C (325°F). Grease a 20 cm (8 in) cake tin and line it with non-stick baking parchment.

Place the cream in a saucepan and bring to a rapid boil. Remove from the heat and cool slightly.

Sift the flour and baking powder together.

Place the eggs and sugar in a bowl and whisk until thick and fluffy. Fold in the flour and half the cream. When thoroughly mixed, add the remaining cream and stir until smooth. Pour the mixture into the cake tin and bake for 30 minutes.

Serve warm with citrus sauce or cream.

Serves 8

Meringue-crusted Peach Flan

CRUST

Preheat the oven to 140°C (275°F). Lightly grease a 20–23 cm (8–9 in) pie plate or flan tin. Dust the bottom and sides with cornflour.

Whisk the egg whites with the lemon juice until they form stiff peaks. Add sugar gradually, a spoonful at a time, beating well after each addition. Spread the meringue across the bottom and up the sides of the pie plate. Bake for 1 hour, then leave to cool.

TO MAKE THE FILLING

Place the peach halves, water and sugar in a saucepan and bring slowly to the boil. Reduce the heat and let the fruit simmer until tender (5–8 minutes).

Remove the fruit from the heat and let it cool, then purée the mixture in a blender or food processor.

Mix the cornflour and sugar with the egg yolks and 2 cups of the peach purée.

INGREDIENTS

CRUST

a little cornflour (cornstarch)

2 egg whites

¼ teaspoon lemon juice

½ cup (125 g, 4 oz) sugar

FILLING

5 fresh peaches

¾ cup (185 mL, 8 fl oz) water

¼ cup (60 g, 2 oz) sugar

2 tablespoons cornflour (cornstarch)

2 tablespoons sugar

2 egg yolks

TOPPING

1 fresh peach, sliced thinly

1 cup (250 mL, 8 fl oz) white wine

3 teaspoons arrowroot

fresh whipped cream, for serving

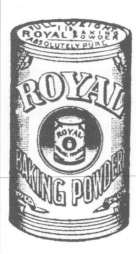

Cook over a medium heat, stirring occasionally, until the mixture boils and thickens. Remove from the heat and continue stirring until cool.

TO ASSEMBLE THE FLAN

Spoon the cooled peach filling into the cooled meringue crust, then return the flan to the refrigerator.

Arrange the thinly sliced peach across the top of the chilled flan. In a small bowl, blend the white wine with the arrowroot. Place this mixture in a small saucepan and cook over a low heat until the mixture boils and thickens. Let the mixture cool slightly, then pour it over the peach slices.

Chill the flan until cold (about 2 hours), then serve with fresh whipped cream.

Serves 6

Sodium-free Baking Powder (Soda)

Combine all ingredients and store in an airtight container.

Use 1 heaped teaspoon per 250 g (8 oz) plain (all-purpose) flour, or 1½ times the normal amount.

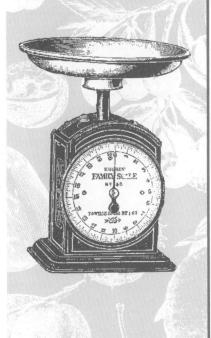

SODIUM-FREE BAKING POWDER

Potassium bicarbonate 39.8 g

Starch 28 g

Tartaric acid 7.5 g

Potassium bitartrate 56.1 g

ORANGE RICE CUSTARD

1 cup (185 g, 6 oz) raw short grain rice

½ cup (125 mL, 4 fl oz) water

1 cup (250 mL, 8 fl oz) single (light, whipping) cream

¼ cup (60 g, 2 oz) sugar

1 cup (250 mL, 8 fl oz) orange juice

⅔ cup (155 mL, 5 fl oz) double (heavy, thickened) cream

zest of 1 orange

sponge fingers (see page 110), for serving

Orange Rice Custard

Place the rice in a double boiler with the water and cream, and steam until the rice is tender (about 1 hour).

Then add the sugar, orange juice and zest to the mixture and stir to combine.

Let the mixture cool.

Place the double cream in a bowl and whip until it forms soft peaks, then fold in the rice mixture. Pour into six parfait glasses and chill for 2 hours before serving.

Serve with sponge fingers.

Serves 6

Salzburg Nockerln

INGREDIENTS

4 egg yolks

2 cups (500 mL, 16 fl oz) milk

1¾ cups (435 g, 14 oz) sugar

30 g (1 oz) plain (all-purpose) flour, sifted

4 egg whites

zest and juice of 2 oranges

Preheat the oven to 180°C (350°F). Lightly grease a 1½ litre (3 pint) pudding bowl or pie dish.

In a bowl, mix the egg yolks and milk together.

In a separate bowl, mix the sugar and flour. Make a well in the centre and pour in the egg yolk and milk mixture.

In a third bowl, whisk the egg whites until they form stiff peaks.

Fold the egg whites into the flour mixture, then add the orange zest and juice.

Pour the mixture into the pudding bowl or pie dish. Place the dish in a baking tray and pour water into the tray so that it reaches halfway up the sides of the dish. Cook the nockerln for 45 minutes.

Let the nockerln cool, then serve it on its own.

Serves 6 to 8

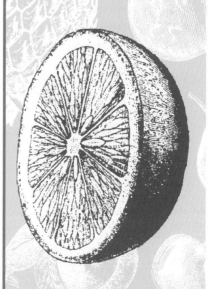

Orange Sesame Seed Cookies

Preheat the oven to 180°C (350°F). Line a baking tray (sheet) with non-stick baking parchment.

Place the sugar and butter in a mixing bowl and whip until light and creamy and pale in colour.

Add the egg and beat well, then add the brandy, lemon zest, flour and sesame seeds.

Mix until a dough is formed. Wrap the dough in plastic wrap (cling film) and refrigerate it for 1 hour. Then roll it out thinly (2 mm, ½ in). Roll the dough out between two sheets of plastic wrap or non-stick baking parchment, as it is soft.

Cut the dough into the desired shapes and bake for 12–15 minutes, or until golden brown around the edges.

Makes 24

INGREDIENTS

ORANGE SESAME SEED COOKIES

½ cup (125 g, 4 oz) sugar

90 g (3 oz) unsalted butter

1 egg

1 tablespoon brandy

zest of 1 lemon

1½ cups (185 g, 6 oz) plain (all-purpose) flour, sifted

3 tablespoons roasted sesame seeds

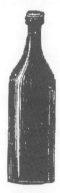

DROP SCONES

125 g (4 oz) unsalted butter

½ cup (125 g, 4 oz) sugar

finely grated zest of 1 lemon

1 egg

1 teaspoon vanilla extract

1 cup (125 g, 4 oz) plain (all-purpose) flour, sifted

1½ teaspoons sodium-free baking powder (soda) (see page 121)

whipped cream and fresh fruit, for serving

Drop Scones

Preheat the oven to 180°C (350°F). Line a baking tray (sheet) with non-stick baking parchment.

Place the butter and sugar in a medium sized bowl and beat until light and fluffy. Add the egg and beat in well.

Add the vanilla, flour and baking powder and stir the mixture until smooth.

Drop heaped spoonfuls of the batter onto the baking tray and bake for 10–15 minutes, or until golden brown.

Serve the drop scones with whipped cream and fresh fruit for a light morning or afternoon tea treat.

Makes 20

Farmhouse Spiced Polenta Pudding

Preheat the oven to 150°C (300°F). Lightly grease or oil a medium sized (2 litre, 3½ imp. pint) baking dish.

In a bowl, combine the polenta, cloves and cinnamon.

Place half the milk in a medium saucepan and bring to the boil. Carefully add the polenta mixture and stir constantly, still over the heat.

Reduce the heat slightly and add the golden syrup, along with the remaining half of the milk. Stir the mixture over a low heat till it is thick. Stir continuously to stop the mixture sticking and burning.

Pour the mixture into the baking dish.

Dot the top of the pudding with teaspoonfuls of the softened butter, then place the baking dish in a large tray of warm water and bake in the water bath for 3 hours.

INGREDIENTS

½ cup (60 g, 2 oz) polenta (cornmeal)

¼ teaspoon ground cloves

½ teaspoon ground cinnamon

2⅔ cups (660 mL, 21 fl oz) milk

¼ cup (90 g, 3 oz) golden syrup (light treacle)

3 teaspoons unsalted butter, softened

double (heavy, thickened) cream or lightly spiced custard, for serving

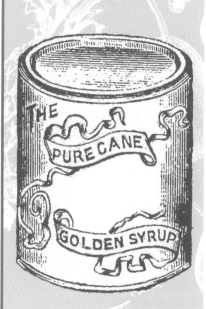

Serve warm with thickened cream or a lightly spiced custard.

Serves 4

Apple Pudding

Peel, core and chop the apples.

Place the apples, water and the first amount of brown sugar in a saucepan and cook over a low heat with the lid on for 15–20 minutes, to reduce the apples to a stewed apple pulp.

Remove the apple mixture from the heat and leave it to cool.

Purée the cooled apple mixture in a blender or food processor. Set aside 375 mL (12 fl oz) of the purée.

Melt the butter in a saucepan, then add the extra brown sugar. Increase the heat slightly and cook, stirring constantly, until the mixture caramelises (2–3 minutes). Stir in the apple purée. Remove the mixture from the heat and let it cool.

5 medium sized green cooking (Granny Smith) apples

100 mL (3½ fl oz) water

2 tablespoons brown sugar (light)

2 tablespoons unsalted butter

½ cup (75 g, 2½ oz) brown sugar (light), extra

1 tablespoon unsalted butter, extra

2 tablespoons sugar

1 cup (125 g, 4 oz) dry breadcrumbs

1 teaspoon ground cinnamon

4 tablespoons thick dairy cream such as clotted cream and sprigs of fresh mint, for serving

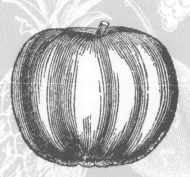

In a frypan (skillet), melt the extra butter over a gentle heat, then stir in the sugar. Let the mixture begin to caramelise slightly, then stir in the breadcrumbs and cinnamon.

Cook the mixture for 1–2 minutes, then remove from the heat and leave to cool completely.

Layer the two mixtures alternately into tall parfait glasses. Top each dessert with a dollop of thickened cream and a sprig of fresh mint.

Serves 4

125

Cardamom Sable Cookies

Preheat the oven to 180°C (350°F). Line a baking tray (sheet) with non-stick baking parchment.

In a bowl, combine the flour, cardamom and sugar. Rub in the butter and lemon zest to form a dough.

Roll the dough into a sausage shape 2 cm (¾ in) thick. Sprinkle the extra sugar evenly over the work surface. Roll the sausage shape in the sugar, then carefully wrap it in plastic wrap (cling film) and freeze it for 2–3 hours.

Remove the dough from the freezer and roll it in the sugar again, then cut it into 3 mm (⅛ in) rounds. Place the rounds on the baking tray and bake for 10–12 minutes, until just turning golden brown.

Remove the cookies from the oven immediately and leave them to cool on the tray.

Makes 24

INGREDIENTS

CARDAMOM SABLE COOKIES

1 cup (125 g, 4 oz) plain (all-purpose) flour, sifted

½ teaspoon ground cardamom

¼ cup (60 g, 2 oz) sugar

125 g (4 oz) unsalted butter, chopped into small pieces

zest of 1 lemon

1 tablespoon sugar, extra

COFFEE MOUSSE

2 teaspoons powdered gelatine

2 tablespoons water

1 tablespoon instant coffee granules

¼ cup (60 mL, 2 fl oz) boiling water

2 tablespoons coffee liqueur (Kahlua)

1⅓ cups (340 mL, 11 fl oz) double (heavy, thickened) cream

⅓ cup (60 g, 2 oz) icing (powdered) sugar

finely grated zest of 1 orange

coffee sauce, or chocolate sauce (see page 102), for serving

Coffee Mousse

Place the gelatine in a small bowl with the first amount of water and leave it to soak for 20–25 minutes.

Dissolve the coffee granules in the boiling water, then add the gelatine. Stir until the gelatine has dissolved.

Stir in the coffee liqueur, then let the mixture cool for 15–20 minutes.

In a bowl, whip the cream with the icing sugar until it forms stiff peaks. Fold in the orange zest and the coffee liquid.

Pour the mixture into a tray 23 x 18 x 3 cm (9 x 7 x 1 in) and chill for 2–3 hours, or until firm.

Cut the mousse into 5 x 5 cm (2 x 2 in) squares and serve on a coffee sauce or with chocolate sauce.

Serves 4

INDEX

Numbers in *italics* indicate photographs

Afternoon Tea Lemon Cake, English 119
Akwadu Pancakes 30
Almandines, Orange *56*, 57
Almond, Apple and Zucchini Cake *18*, 19
Almond Bread *93*, 95
Almond Cinnamon Flan *73*, 80
Almond Torte, Moist 78
Angel Food Cake 54, *55*
Apple, Cheese and Coconut Delight 45
Apple, Raspberry and Apricot Puddings 66
Apple and Apricot Torte 117
Apple Cake, with Almond and Zucchini
  18, 19
Apple Cookies *35*, 42
Apple Fritters 12
Apple Pudding 125
Apple Upside Down Cake 84
Apples, Baked 48
Apricot and Apple Torte 117
Apricot and Hazelnut Meringue Slice 34, *35*
Apricot Mousse with a Symphony of
  Sauces *37*, 39
Apricot, Orange and Yoghurt Mousse 25
Apricot Puddings, with Apple and
  Raspberry 66
Apricot Whip 61
Baked Apples 48
Baked Cheesecake 77
Baking Powder, Sodium-free 121
Banana and Cinnamon Soufflé 60
Bavarois, Split Berry *38*, 53
Beetroot Cake 101
Berries, Marinated, with Blackberry Pots 27
Berry (Split) Bavarois *38*, 53
Berry and Cheesy Filo Stacks 16
Berry and Mango Brulée 10
Berry Soufflé 79
Biscuits
  Apple Sauce *35*
Bitter Marmalade Cake 99
Black Bun, Scotch 119
Blackberry Tart, Creamy 87
Blackberry Pots with Marinated Berries 27
Blueberry Pie 103
Blueberry Pies, Individual 47
Boiled Fruit Cake 104
Bread
  Almond *93*, 95
  Carrot and Cardamom 21
  Glazed Spicy Fruit Loaf 90

Scotch Black Bun 119
  Spiced Coffee 68
  Sweet Loaf 59
Bread Rolls, Sweet or Savoury 105
Brownies
  Chocolate 20
  Deluxe Chocolate 40
Brulée
  Berry and Mango 10
  Pumpkin and Raspberry 63
Bun, Scotch Black 119
Buns, Sweet Bread 59
Butter, Lemon 42
Cake
  Almond, Apple and Zucchini *18*, 19
  Angel Food 54, *55*
  Apple Upside Down 84
  Baked Cheesecake 77
  Beetroot 101
  Bitter Marmalade 99
  Boiled Fruit 104
  Chocolate 14
  Chocolate (Flourless) 85
  Cornflour Sponge 80
  English Afternoon Tea Lemon 119
  Fruit 76
  Josef 69
  Lemon and Cardamom Syrup *36*, 40
  Light Lemon 15
  Luscious Coconut Cream 83
  Pear 107
  Sienna 11
  Walnut (Flourless) 100
  Wholemeal Spice and Lemon 104
Cardamom and Carrot Bread 21
Cardamom and Lemon Syrup Cake *36*, 40
Cardamom Sable Cookies 126
Carrot and Cardamom Bread 21
Cheese, Apple and Coconut Delight 45
Cheesecake
  Baked 77
  Raspberry 86
Cheesy Filo and Berry Stacks 16, *17*
Cherry Soup 116
Chocolate and Orange Muffins 82
Chocolate Brownies 20
Chocolate Brownies, Deluxe 40
Chocolate Cake 14
Chocolate Cake (Flourless) 85
Chocolate Chip Muffins 101

Chocolate Mocha Custards 110, *111*
Chocolate Mousse Torte *74*, 75
Chocolate Peanut Butter Cookies 44
Chocolate Sauce 102
Cinnamon Almond Flan *73*, 80
Cinnamon and Lemon Cookies 49
Cinnamon and Banana Soufflé 60
Cinnamon Orange Crisps 20
Citrus Crumble 84
Citrus Jellies, with Sauterne *92*, 97
Citrus Puddings 48
Citrus Salad, Gluhwein-marinated 62
Citrus Sauce 64
Citrus Soufflé, Frozen 32
Clove Cookies, Mediterranean *93*, 96
Coconut Cream Cake, Luscious 83
Coconut Delight, with Apple and Cheese 45
Coconut Macaroons 82
Coffee Bread, Spiced 68
Coffee Mousse 126
Cookies
  Apple *35*, 42
  Cardamom Sable 126
  Chocolate Peanut Butter 44
  Lemon and Cinnamon 49
  Mediterranean Clove *93*, 96
  Orange Sesame Seed 123
Cornflour Sponge 80
Cream, Raspberry Polenta 81
Creamy Blackberry Tart 87
Crème de la Coeur 58
Crumble, Citrus 84
Crumble-topped Honey Pears 12
Custard
  Chocolate Mocha 110, *111*
  Orange Rice 121
  Vanilla 30
Deluxe Chocolate Brownies 40
Drop Scones 123
Drunken Plums 54
Eggs, Snow 59
English Afternoon Tea Lemon Cake 119
English Breakfast Marmalade 43
English Rice Pudding Tropical 76
Farmhouse Spiced Polenta Pudding 124
Figgy Pudding, Steamed 22
Figs, Pickled *18*, 19
Fingers, Sponge 110, *111*
Flan
  Cinnamon Almond *73*, 80

Meringue-crusted Peach 120
Flourless Chocolate Cake 85
Flourless Walnut Cake 100
Fritters, Apple 12
Frozen Citrus Soufflé 32
Fruit Cake 76
Fruit Cake, Boiled 104
Fruit Loaf, Spicy (Glazed) 90
Fruit Pancake Stack 118
Fruit Pie, 'Snow Top' 26
Fruit Pudding, Steamed 106
Fruit Sensation 46
Gelato 102
Glazed Spicy Fruit Loaf 90
Gluhwein-marinated Citrus Salad 62
Hazelnut and Apricot Meringue Slice 34, 35
Honey Slice 91, 98
Ice Cream, Pumpkin 44
Ice Cream 33
Individual Blueberry Pies 47
Japonaise Torte 72
Jellies, Sauterne and Citrus 92, 97
Josef Cake 69
Kisses, Meringue 112, 113
Koshav, Polish Sweet 51
Lemon and Cardamom Syrup Cake 36, 40
Lemon and Cinnamon Cookies 49
Lemon and Spice Cake, Wholemeal 104
Lemon and Sultana Muffins, Wholemeal
  56, 57
Lemon Butter 42
Lemon Cake, English Afternoon Tea 119
Lemon Cake, Light 15
Lemon Curd Pots 73, 81
Lemon Snow 107
Lemon Torte, Zesty 52
Light Lemon Cake 15
Light Tropical Roll 38, 67
Luscious Coconut Cream Cake 83
Macaroons, Coconut 82
Mango and Berry Brulée 10
Marmalade, English Breakfast 43
Marmalade (Bitter) Cake 99
Mediterranean Clove Cookies 93, 96
Meringue Kisses 112, 113
Meringue Slice, Apricot and Hazelnut 34, 35
Meringue-crusted Peach Flan 120
Mocha and Chocolate Custard 110, 111
Moist Almond Torte 78
Mousse
  Apricot, with a Symphony of Sauces 37,
  39
  Chocolate, Torte 74, 75
  Coffee 126
  Yoghurt, Apricot and Orange 25
Muffins
  Chocolate Chip 101
  Orange Chocolate 82
  Lemon and Sultana, Wholemeal 56, 57
  Raspberry 13
  Sour Cream and Peanut 94, 113

Nockerln, Salzburg 122
Orange Almandines 56, 57
Orange, Apricot and Yoghurt Mousse 25
Orange Chocolate Muffins 82
Orange Cinnamon Crisps 20
Orange Rice Custard 121
Orange Sesame Seed Cookies 123
Pancake Fruit Stack 118
Pancakes, Akwadu 30
Parfaits, Pomegranate 24
Passionfruit Soufflé 24
Pavlova 75
Peach Flan, Meringue-crusted 120
Peanut and Sour Cream Muffins 94, 113
Peanut Butter and Chocolate Cookies 44
Pear Cake 107
Pears, Crumble-topped Honey 12
Pie
  Blueberry 103
  Individual Blueberry 47
  'Snow Top' Fruit 26
Pickled Figs 18, 19
Plums, Drunken 54
Polenta Cream, Raspberry 81
Polenta Pudding, Farmhouse Spiced 124
Polish Sweet Koshav 51
Pomegranate Parfaits 24
Pots
  Blackberry, with Marinated Berries 27
  Lemon Curd 73, 81
Pudding
  Apple 125
  Apple, Apricot and Raspberry 66
  Apricot, with Apple and Raspberry 66
  Citrus 48
  Farmhouse Spiced Polenta 124
  Steamed Figgy 22
  Steamed Fruit 106
  Summer 23
  Tropical English Rice 76
Pumpkin and Raspberry Brulées 63
Pumpkin Ice Cream 44
Raspberry and Apple, with Apricot
  Puddings 66
Raspberry and Pumpkin Brulées 63
Raspberry Cheesecake 86
Raspberry Divinity 65
Raspberry Muffins 13
Raspberry Polenta Cream 81
Raspberry Pudding, with Apple and
  Apricot 66
Raspberry Sorbet 112, 114
Rice Custard, Orange 121
Rice Pudding, Tropical English 76
Roll, Light Tropical 38, 67
Sable Cookies, Cardamom 126
Salad, Citrus, Gluhwein-marinated 62
Salzburg Nockerln 122
Sauce
  Chocolate 102
  Citrus 64

Sauterne and Citrus Jellies 92, 97
Savoury or Sweet Bread Rolls 105
Scones, Drop 123
Scotch Black Bun 119
Sesame Seed and Orange Cookies 123
Sherbet, Strawberry 45
Shortbread 115
Sienna Cake 11
Slice
  Apricot and Hazelnut Meringue 34, 35
  Honey 91, 98
'Snow Top' Fruit Pie 26
Snow, Lemon 107
Snow Eggs 59
Sodium-free Baking Powder 121
Sorbet, Raspberry 112, 114
Soufflé
  Banana and Cinnamon 60
  Berry 79 .
  Frozen Citrus 32
  Passionfruit 24
Soup, Cherry 116
Sour Cream and Peanut Muffins 94, 113
Spice and Lemon Cake, Wholemeal 104
Spiced Coffee Bread 68
Spiced Polenta Pudding, Farmhouse 124
Spicy Fruit Loaf, Glazed 90
Split Berry Bavarois 38, 53
Sponge, Cornflour 80
Sponge Fingers 110, 111
Steamed Figgy Pudding 22
Steamed Fruit Pudding 106
Strawberry Sherbet 45
Sultana and Lemon Muffins, Wholemeal
  56, 57
Summer Pudding 23
Sweet Bread Buns 59
Sweet or Savoury Bread Rolls 105
Tart
  Creamy Blackberry 87
Torte
  Apple and Apricot 117
  Chocolate Mousse 74, 75
  Japonaise 72
  Moist Almond 78
  Zesty Lemon 52
Tropical English Rice Pudding 76
Tropical Roll, Light 38, 67
Vanilla Custards 30
Walnut Cake, Flourless 100
Whip, Apricot 61
Wholemeal Lemon and Sultana Muffins 56,
  57
Wholemeal Spice and Lemon Cake 104
Yoghurt, Apricot and Oranage Mousse 25
Yoghurt Mousse, Apricot, with a Symph-
  ony of Sauces (2)
Zabaglione 93, 97
Zesty Lemon Torte 52
Zucchini Cake, with Almond and Apple
  18, 19